The Integrative Herbalist

Earth, Alchemy, and Embodied Plant Medicine

Dr. Stephanie Shelburne

with

New England School of Bioenergetic Medicine

Three Pools Publishing

The Integrative Herbalist: Earth, Alchemy, and Embodied Plant Medicine

Library of Congress Cataloguing-in-Publication Data

Shelburne, Dr. Stephanie

The Integrative Herbalist: Earth, Alchemy, and Embodied Plant Medicine / Dr. Stephanie Shelburne

ISBN-13: 978-1-968683-99-3 (Paperback. 2026)

ISBN-13: 978-1-968683-93-1 (Ebook. 2026)

Three Pools Publishing

PO Box 74

North Adam, Massachusetts

www.ThreePoolsPublishing.com

Contents

For the plants themselves,
who have been teaching since before there were students.
For those who tend the old ways
and for those just beginning to remember.
For the land that holds us
and the generations yet to come.

A Note from the Author

I am finalizing this body of work from a farmhouse in Vermont, now surrounded by snow but remembering, that underneath the cold white landscape, I am surrounded by the plants who have become my teachers, my companions, my kin over these past few years.

In my mind's eye, I remember the garden where nettles and chamomile grow alongside vegetables, where calendula self-seeds in cheerful orange abundance, where the mint has escaped its bounds (as mint always does) and colonized the edges of everything. Beyond the garden, the forest holds its own pharmacy - black cohosh in the understory, wild raspberry along the edges, reishi on the fallen oaks. This and other landscapes have been teaching me for years, and I recognize that I am still very much a student.

This book has been a decade in the making, emerging piece by piece, from a simple recognition: the way we typically teach herbalism is incomplete. We teach constituents and actions, protocols and contraindications - all necessary, all valuable. But we often forget to teach relationship. We forget that the plants are not passive resources waiting to be used but living intelligences offering to meet us, if we know how to approach them. We forget that the body is not a machine to be fixed but a wisdom to be partnered with. We forget that healing is not something we do *to* people but something that happens *between* - between plant and person, between practitioner and client, between the visible and the invisible forces that shape our lives.

I have spent my professional life in the space between worlds - between Western science and traditional wisdom, between the measurable and the mysterious, between the clinical and the sacred. My training includes the languages of research and physiology, the frameworks of functional medicine and clinical nutrition. But my deepest teachers have been the rhythms of the seasons, the wisdom of my own body, the ancient lineages that understood healing as participation in something larger than ourselves, and the natural world itself.

This book attempts to hold both: the rigor of integrative science and the depth of embodied, relational practice. I have not tried to strip away the mystery in favor of mechanism, nor to abandon the value of research in favor of romance. Both are needed. The herbalist who understands liver biochemistry, can sense the quality of imbalance in a person's energy, *and* engage deeply in conversation with the plant world is the herbalist who can truly serve.

The title speaks of three things: Earth, Alchemy, and Embodied Plant Medicine.

Earth because all of this begins and ends with the living planet - the soil that grows the plants, the seasons that time our work, the ecosystems we must protect if there is to be plant medicine for future generations. Without healthy earth, there are no herbs. Without reciprocity with the land, our practice becomes extraction rather than relationship.

Alchemy because this journey is, at its heart, alchemical - elemental and primal. The transformation of plant into medicine follows the same archetypal pattern that the alchemists mapped centuries ago: the breaking down of raw material, the purification through various stages, the recombination into something more potent than the original. Fire, water, earth, air - the classical elements are not metaphors here but actual forces you will work with. You will use water to draw out the water-soluble gifts of plants. You will use alcohol - fire captured in liquid form - to extract what water cannot reach. You will work with the earth of roots and the air of aromatics. This is elemental work, primal work, hands in the soil and fire under the pot.

And the alchemists understood what modern medicine often forgets: the practitioner is transformed alongside the substance. You cannot do this work without being changed by it. The *opus* - the great work - acts on the operator as surely as on the material. The *nigredo* of unknowing gives way to the *albedo* of purification through study, which yields to the *citrinitas* of dawning understanding, which culminates in the *rubedo* - the reddening, the completion, the emergence of gold. By the end of this book, you will not only know more; you will *be* more. You will have become an alchemist.

Embodied because this is not abstract knowledge to store in the mind but lived wisdom to know in the body. Every chapter includes practices that ask you to taste, to feel, to sense, to make. You will not merely read about herbs; you will meet them directly, prepare them with your own hands, take them into your own body, observe their effects. This knowing cannot be transmitted through words alone. It must be lived.

I have organized this book as a journey - an alchemical passage that mirrors both the traditional apprenticeship and the stages of the great work itself. You will begin with the foundations: the relationship with plants, the language of energetics, the primal skills of preparation. This is the *prima materia* - the raw material from which everything else will be refined. Then you will move through the wheel of the year with its seasonal wisdoms, through the lunar rhythms that pattern plant and body alike - learning to work with elemental time, with the forces that govern growth and rest, accumulation and release. Finally, you will enter the alchemist's laboratory, learning to create formulas from the meeting of plant intelligence with human need, stepping into your identity as one who transforms.

The structure is not arbitrary. It mirrors the alchemical stages: dissolution, purification, recombination, completion. Each phase builds on what came before. A note about the seasonal quality highlighted within, remember also that seasons are reflected in our daily lives, across the spectrum of our lived trajectory. Winter is not only the regenerative time of the year, but also of the day/night, and of the waxing and waning of the years of our life. As such, the seasonal chapters of this text are an expression of multidimensionality.

A word about what this book is not. It is not a comprehensive materia medica - there are excellent ones already, and the best one is the one you will build yourself from your own experience. It is not a medical text or a substitute for professional diagnosis and treatment. It is not, in fact, the final word on anything; rather it is an invitation into ongoing relationship with plants, with bodies, with the mystery of healing itself. Consider it a doorway rather than a destination.

I write as someone who believes that the world needs more people who know plants - not just academically, but relationally. People who can make medicine, who can read bodies, who can tend the sick with wisdom and humility. People who remember that humans and plants have been in partnership since the beginning, and who are willing to continue that partnership into whatever future we are creating together. If you are called to be such a person, this book is for you.

The plants are waiting. They have been waiting a long time. Perhaps they have been waiting for you.

With gratitude for the natural world,
Stephanie
Vermont, in the season of deep rest

Introduction

The Forgotten Partnership

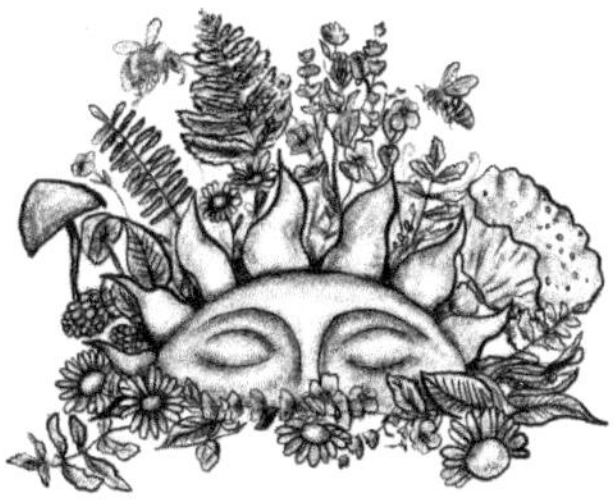

For most of human history, we knew the plants. Not as abstractions in a textbook or products on a shelf, but as neighbors, as presences, as beings with whom we shared the world. We knew which ones could feed us and which could kill us, which could ease a fever and which could open visions, which could help a mother's milk flow, and which could stop a wound from bleeding. This knowledge was not separate from daily life but woven through it - passed from grandmother to grandchild, from healer to apprentice, from the plants themselves to anyone willing to pay attention.

This was primal knowledge - knowledge held in the body, in the senses, in the hands that gathered and prepared. It was elemental work: fire under the cauldron, water drawing out medicine, earth yielding roots, air carrying the scent of drying herbs. Our ancestors did not need to call it alchemy; they simply lived it, participated in the eternal dance of transformation that turns plant into medicine, medicine into healing, healing into wholeness.

Something has been lost. Not entirely - the knowledge persists in pockets, in lineages, in the stubborn memory of bodies that still respond to chamomile and peppermint even when the mind has forgotten why. But for most people in the modern world, the relationship has been severed. Plants have become ingredients, commodities, decorations. Medicine has become something manufactured in factories, dispensed by professionals, swallowed without understanding. The living partnership between humans and the green world has faded into a faint cultural memory, a nostalgic image of grandmothers and gardens that seems to have little relevance to contemporary life.

And yet. Something is stirring. People are returning to plants - not as regression to a simpler past, but as reclamation of something essential that never should have been abandoned. They are planting gardens, making tinctures, learning the names of what grows around them. They are questioning a medical system that often treats symptoms while ignoring causes, that offers pharmaceuticals for every complaint while the underlying patterns of imbalance persist. They are seeking a different relationship with their own bodies - not as machines to be managed by experts but as intelligent living systems with their own wisdom about what they need.

This book is for those people. It is for anyone who has feels the call to know plants more deeply - whether you dream of becoming a clinical herbalist or simply want to care for yourself and your family with more wisdom, or are drawn to plants for reasons you can't quite articulate but feel in your bones. It is for those who sense that healing is more than chemistry, that bodies are more than mechanisms, that the world is more alive and interconnected than the dominant culture admits.

THE ALCHEMICAL JOURNEY

This book will lead you on a journey that is both ancient and immediate - an alchemical passage through the elements, through the seasons, through the transformation of self and substance. It is primal work, rooted in the body and the senses, grounded in direct experience rather than abstract theory. And it will change you, as all true alchemical work changes the one who undertakes it.

You will learn to see plants differently - not as static objects but as living beings with their own intelligence, their own personalities, their own gifts to offer. You will learn to approach them in relationship rather than extraction, to ask before taking, to give back as well as receive. This is not sentimentality; it is the foundation on which effective herbal practice is built. The herbalist who knows plants as allies creates better medicine than the one who knows them only as ingredients.

You will learn the language of energetics - the traditional understanding of hot and cold, dry and damp, tense and lax that allows you to match plant to person with precision. These are elemental qualities: fire's heat and water's coolness, air's dryness and earth's moisture. Modern herbalism often neglects this language in favor of standardized protocols, but the traditional approach remains powerful: it sees each person as unique, each pattern of imbalance as specific, each herbal intervention as a conversation between the qualities of the plant and the needs of the person.

You will learn to read bodies - to recognize the signs of tissue states, the patterns of excess and deficiency, the constitutional tendencies that shape how each person experiences health and illness. This is clinical thinking, but not the reductive kind that sees only diagnoses and treatment protocols. It is a holistic reading that considers the whole person: body, mind, emotions, spirit, and the circumstances of their life.

You will journey through the wheel of the year, learning how each season offers its own wisdom for health and its own herbal allies. Spring's rising energy and its support for clearing and renewal. Summer's fullness and its care for the systems that protect and circulate. Autumn's gathering and its nourishment of nervous system and structure. Winter's deep rest and its attention to reproduction, restoration, and the reserves we draw upon in hard times. You will follow the moon through her phases, learning the celestial rhythms that pattern plant and body alike. This is elemental time - not the mechanical tick of clocks but the living pulse of a planet dancing with sun and moon.

You will learn the art of formulation - how to combine individual herbs into complex medicines that address the whole pattern of a person's imbalance. This is where herbalism becomes truly sophisticated, where you learn to create remedies that are greater than the sum of their parts. It is also where you step fully into the role of alchemist, working with the primal forces of transformation to create medicines tailored to the unique person before you.

And through all of this, you will be transformed. This is perhaps the most important teaching, and the one least often spoken: the study of plant medicine changes the one who studies. You will develop new senses, new ways of perceiving, new capacities for attention. You will begin to feel yourself as part of the web of life rather than separate from it. You will become, in some measure, what you are learning - more grounded, more attuned, more able to be present with suffering and participate in healing. The plants will work on you even as you learn to work with them. This is the alchemist's secret: you cannot transform the substance without being transformed yourself.

How to Use This Book

This book is organized as a journey, and I encourage you to take it as one. Begin at the beginning. Don't skip ahead to the formulation chapters before you've absorbed the foundations of energetics and the seasonal wisdom. Each section builds on what came before; the later material will make more sense and land more deeply if you've done the earlier work.

Every chapter ends with an embodied practice - something to do, not just to read. These practices are essential. You cannot learn herbalism from a book; you can only learn it from plants, from bodies, from direct experience. The book offers maps and guidance, but you must walk the territory yourself. Make the medicines. Taste the herbs. Do the practices. Your body is as much a student as your mind, and some things can only be learned through the hands, the tongue, the senses.

Keep a journal as you go. Record your experiences with each herb you meet - what you tasted, what you felt, what you observed. Record the formulas you create and their effects. Record your questions and confusions as well as your insights. This journal will become the beginning of your own materia medica, your personal record of relationship with the green world. Years from now, you will look back at it and see how far you've traveled.

Be patient with yourself. Learning herbalism is not a matter of memorizing information; it is a matter of developing relationship, building capacity, allowing transformation. This takes time. Some things will click immediately; others will take months or years to fully understand. Trust the process. The plants are patient teachers; let yourself be a patient student.

On Professionalism and Scope of Practice

Herbs are powerful. This is precisely why they can help - and also why they must be used with knowledge and respect. Throughout this book, I offer safety information, contraindications, and cautions. Take them seriously. This is part of what it means to practice with integrity.

I want to speak directly about something that is often handled clumsily in herbal education: the question of professional standing and referral. If you study with rigor, develop real competence, and practice with integrity, you *are* a professional. You deserve to be recognized as such. The trained herbalist who has done the deep work of learning plants, understanding bodies, and developing clinical skill is not an amateur playing at healing; they are a practitioner of one of humanity's oldest and most sophisticated healing arts.

When we talk about "professional diagnosis," what we are really talking about is scope of practice. Every healing profession has a scope - a domain of competence, a range of conditions and interventions appropriate to that training. Physicians have their scope. Acupuncturists have theirs. Psychotherapists have theirs. And herbalists have theirs. These scopes overlap in places and diverge in others. No single practitioner, regardless of their credentials, can appropriately address every human health concern.

Recognizing your scope of practice - knowing what you can appropriately address and where the boundaries of your competence lie - is not a mark of inadequacy. It is a mark of professionalism. Referring someone to a physician, or to a mental health professional, or to any other practitioner whose scope better fits the person's needs, does not make you less of a professional. It makes you an integrity-rich practitioner. It demonstrates that you care more about the person's wellbeing than about your own ego or income. This kind of ethical awareness is what distinguishes true professionals from those merely playing a role.

Humility, awareness, and ethics all compel us to recognize our scope. The best practitioners - in any field - are those who know what they know, know what they don't know, and act accordingly. They collaborate rather than compete. They refer when referral serves. They remain students even as they become teachers. This is the professionalism I hope you will embody.

Nothing in this book is intended as medical advice for specific conditions. I am offering education in the traditional art of herbalism - rigorous, substantive education that can form the foundation of genuine professional practice. How you use this education, and how you integrate it with other forms of care, is your responsibility. Use it wisely, practice with integrity, and never hesitate to collaborate with or refer to other practitioners when that best serves the person before you.

The Invitation

You are being invited into a very old story - the story of humans and plants, intertwined since the beginning, still unfolding, still needing people willing to carry it forward. This is elemental work, primal work. It will ask you to use your hands, your senses, your body's own intelligence. It will connect you to forces older than civilization - the turning of seasons, the pull of the moon, the alchemy of transformation that has been happening since life began. The plants have been holding up their end of the partnership all along, offering their medicine, waiting for us to remember. The question is whether we will accept the invitation.

This is not about returning to some idealized past. It is about bringing the wisdom of that past into the present, allowing it to evolve, letting it meet the challenges of our time. The herbalism we need now is not identical to what our ancestors practiced; it is informed by their wisdom but also by modern research, by contemporary understandings of physiology and pathology, by the specific conditions of life in this moment. We honor the lineage not by repeating it unchanged but by keeping it alive, adapting it, adding our own learning to what was passed down. The alchemy continues. The elements remain. The primal forces still flow through every plant, every body, every act of healing.

If you have read this far, something in you is saying yes. Trust that. The call to learn plants is itself a kind of guidance - the plants calling to those they want to work with, the lineage reaching for those who will carry it forward, the primal intelligence in your own body recognizing what it needs to remember. You don't need to know yet where this path leads or what kind of herbalist you will become. You only need to take the next step.

The journey begins with the first herb you truly meet, the first medicine you make with your own hands, the first time you taste a plant and feel it teaching you something no book could convey. Fire, water, earth, air - you will work with all of them. Darkness and light, waxing and waning, growth and rest - you will learn their rhythms. And somewhere along the way, the transformation will happen. The alchemist will emerge. It continues for a lifetime - deepening, expanding, revealing new mysteries just when you thought you understood.

Welcome to the path. Welcome to the alchemy.

Part One
Foundations

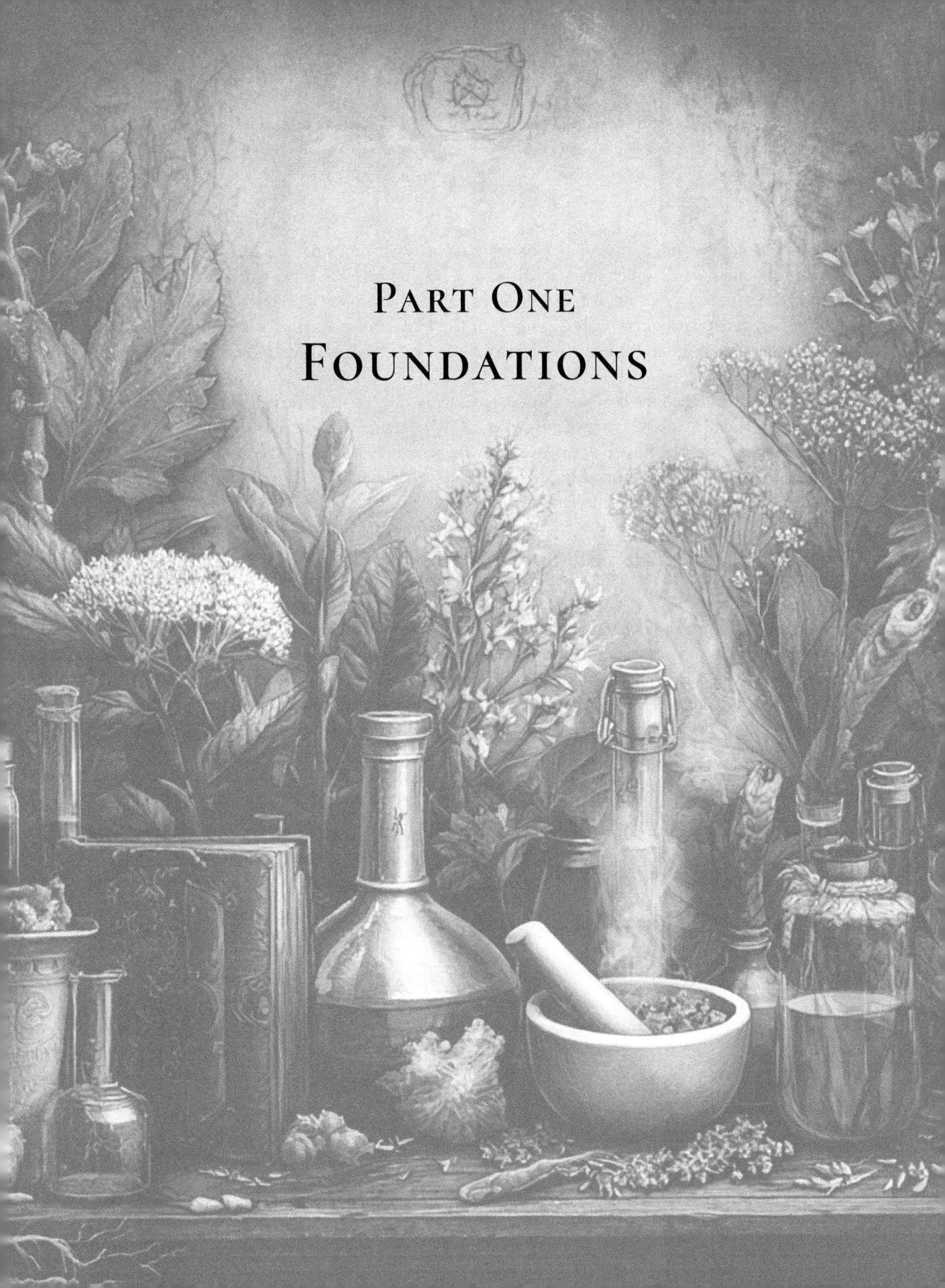

CROSSING THE THRESHOLD INTO RELATIONSHIP

Every journey begins with a threshold - a moment of crossing from what was into what will be. You stand at that threshold now. Behind you lies the world as you have known it, where plants were background, decoration, ingredient. Before you lies a world where plants are teachers, allies, kin. The crossing changes everything, though you may not feel it yet. Some thresholds announce themselves with thunder; others are recognized only in retrospect, when you look back and realize: "Ah yes, that was when it began".

The alchemists called the beginning of the great work the *nigredo* - the blackening, the necessary darkness before dawn. It is the stage of not-yet-knowing, of standing in the fertile void where transformation becomes possible. You do not need to know where this path leads. You do not need to see the whole journey before taking the first step. You need only be willing to cross - to leave behind certainty, to enter relationship, to let the plants begin their work on you.

In the chapters that follow, you will gather the *prima materia* - the raw materials from which everything else will be refined. You will learn to see plants as living intelligences offering relationship rather than resources waiting to be used. You will develop the language of energetics - hot and cold, dry and damp, tense and lax - that allows plant and person to speak to one another across the boundary of species. You will learn the alchemical arts of preparation: how water and alcohol and heat and time transform crude plant matter into refined medicine. And you will begin to read the body's own language, the tissue states and patterns that reveal what each person needs.

This is foundational work - not glamorous, not yet clinical, but essential. A house built on sand will not stand; an herbalist built on shallow understanding will not serve. Take your time with these chapters. Let the concepts sink below the surface of the mind into the knowing of the body. Practice the practices. Taste the herbs. Begin building relationships that will deepen over years and decades of work.

The threshold asks only one thing of you: that you cross it. Not perfectly, not with complete understanding, not without fear or doubt. Just that you step forward, leaving behind the one who did not yet know the plants, becoming - step by step, herb by herb, preparation by preparation - the one who does.

The plants are waiting on the other side. They have been waiting a long time. Cross over, and let the transformation begin.

Chapter 1
Crossing the Threshold
Meeting Plants as Sovereign Beings

Welcome to the Threshold

And here you are.

Behind you is the world where plants are scenery, ingredients, resources - green wallpaper in the background of human life. Ahead is a world where plants are teachers, companions, sovereign beings with whom you can build relationship. Where the rustle of leaves might carry meaning. Where a root offered in tincture is a gift exchanged, not a commodity consumed.

This chapter supports your first steps by providing context, history, and foundation for the journey you're beginning. Read it slowly. Let it settle into your bones. Return to it throughout the module - it will mean different things as you change.

Why Herbs? Why Now?

We all have stories about how herbs seem to slowly unfurl into our lives. For so many of us, it begins the same way - a quiet invitation we almost miss.

Perhaps you had eczema that didn't clear until you tried a burdock tincture from the health food store, and something in you wondered: *how did that work?* Maybe your grandmother's garden held secrets she never quite explained. Perhaps a friend tends her family with herbs grown in her backyard, and you've noticed how differently she moves through illness - not fighting it, but conversing with it. Or you stumbled upon a book about herbal medicine and couldn't put it down, as if it were written for a part of you that had been waiting.

Whatever the reason, when we begin learning about plants, we find ourselves changing in unexpected ways. We may start eating more thoughtfully, reconsidering what we put in and on our bodies, moving with more awareness toward our land and water. We begin noticing things we never saw before - the plantain growing in dusty urban lots, the mugwort along country roadways, the world of medicine growing unbidden at our feet.

Walking in the woods becomes a different experience when you can greet the plants growing around you by name. Not because naming gives you power over them, but because names are how relationship begins.

Why herbs?

Because they work - gently and effectively. Because you can grow many yourself, right outside your front door or even in your kitchen. Because learning herbal medicine connects you to thousands of years of human wisdom and to the living earth itself. Because plants and herbs have sustained the health and well-being of humankind for tens of thousands of years - our nourishment, medicine, shelter, clothing, and in many cultures, our spiritual guides. Our very survival has depended upon our intimate relationship with the plant world.

Our very humanness depends on them, and in return, they depend on us. To deny this is to deny our part in the great web of life. Their out-breath is our in-breath. They feed, clothe, and house us. We are woven into the same interwoven strand.

This is not poetry. This is biology, ecology, truth. You cannot survive without plants. Neither can any other animal. Learning herbalism is, in part, remembering this fundamental relationship - not as concept, but as lived reality.

What Are Herbs?

The botanical definition is straightforward: a plant without a woody stem that bears seeds and dies back after blooming. But in herbalism, we use the term more broadly - any plant used for food, medicine, or sacred purpose. Trees, shrubs, mushrooms, seaweeds - all can be "herbs" in the herbalist's vocabulary.

Here is what matters more than definition: an herb is a being you are entering into relationship with. A chemistry, yes - constituents and actions we can name and study. But also a presence. An intelligence. A teacher with something to offer, if you learn to listen.

Herbalism is sometimes mistakenly grouped with homeopathy, but they are entirely different systems. Homeopathy, founded in the late 18th century, uses minute doses of substances based on the principle of "like cures like." Herbalism, by contrast, is one of the oldest healing traditions known to humanity, using plants themselves as medicine - their actual physical substance, their chemistry and spirit working together.

The Ancient Roots of Herbal Medicine

Herbal medicine represents one of the earliest forms of healthcare practiced by humanity. This tradition spans thousands of years, connecting cultures across continents and time periods in a great web of green wisdom.

Ancient texts preserve fragments of this knowledge. The Sumerian clay tablets from around 3000-2500 BCE are regarded as the oldest written evidence of medicinal plant usage - imagine, someone pressing stylus to clay to record which plants healed which ailments, so the knowledge would not be lost. The Ebers Papyrus of Egypt, from around 1550 BCE, documents hundreds of plant medicines. The Ayurvedic texts of India, dating back over 3,000 years, detail elaborate systems of herbal healing. The Shen Nong Ben Cao Jing, an ancient Chinese pharmacopoeia, describes hundreds of medicinal substances. Indigenous peoples on every continent developed sophisticated knowledge of their local plant medicines, passed through generations in ways we are only beginning to appreciate.

Across centuries, methods for preparing, utilizing, and studying medicinal plants have evolved - shaped by culture, need, and what we call progress.

But how did humans first learn the healing power of plants? The theory most comfortable to the modern mind suggests trial and error - observing sick animals, noticing which plants grew in rich soil, tasting cautiously and watching what happened.

Yet if you've ever truly sat with a plant - not studied it, but *befriended* it - this theory feels not quite right. Plausible, perhaps, to a mind that trusts only the measurable. But insufficient to anyone who has felt a plant reach back.

Our ancestors, I believe, were quantum people. In that connection - that unbroken conversation with the living world - they received guidance. From plants. From animals. From the land itself.

Every ancient culture carries these stories. And yet Western thought dismisses them as charming mythology, preferring the image of our ancestors stumbling behind animals, hoping for the best.

What if the old stories are truer than the theories?

Some cultures eventually organized their observations of seasonal cycles, the elements, plants, and animals into elaborate systems that could be more readily passed on to future generations - like Ayurveda or Traditional Chinese Medicine. Others maintained oral traditions, passing knowledge through story, song, and direct teaching from elder to apprentice. Both paths carry wisdom. Both have something to offer us now.

Herbal Traditions Across Cultures

All over the world, countless herbal traditions blossomed independently, each uniquely shaped by its bioregion's indigenous plants, climate, and cultural wisdom. These are not simply different "systems" of medicine. They are different ways of being in relationship with the green world - different languages for the same ancient conversation.

❧ Ayurveda: The Science of Life

Derived from Sanskrit, "Ayurveda" translates to "science of life." This comprehensive system of medicine originated in India over 5,000 years ago and remains vibrantly practiced today - not as a relic, but as living wisdom that continues to evolve.

Central to the Ayurvedic framework is the understanding that medicinal plants have personalities - properties, therapeutic affinities, and ways of moving through the body that can be learned and mapped. This intricate system classifies herbs according to taste (*rasa*), energy (*virya*), post-digestive effect (*vipaka*), and special potency (*prabhava*). These are not merely intellectual categories - they are ways of knowing plants through direct experience.

The philosophy emphasizes balance among three *doshas* - Vata, Pitta, and Kapha - fundamental energies that govern physiological and psychological functions. Herbal treatments are tailored to restore equilibrium unique to each individual. This is medicine that sees *you*, not just your symptoms.

❧ Traditional Chinese Medicine

Traditional Chinese Medicine represents one of the oldest healing systems globally, with roots extending over 2,500 years. Centered on the concept of achieving balance within the body, TCM employs a holistic framework integrating Qi (vital energy), Yin and Yang, and the Five Elements theory.

The sophistication of TCM herbal medicine lies in its formulas - tailored to each individual's unique constitution and health concerns, combining herbs that work synergistically rather than in isolation. Where Western pharmacology often seeks to isolate single active compounds, TCM recognizes that plants are communities of chemistry, and that removing a plant from its wholeness may also remove its wisdom.

This is a tradition that has watched herbs work in human bodies for millennia. That kind of observation carries weight.

❧ European Herbalism

The European herbal tradition as we know it draws from Greek, Roman, and Celtic wisdom - but what we know is only what survived.

Hippocrates, called the "Father of Medicine," taught that healing flows from nature herself. Dioscorides, a Greek physician of the 1st century CE, compiled *De Materia Medica*, describing over 600 plants in a text that would guide healers for fifteen centuries. These names anchor our history.

During the Renaissance, herbals became some of the first printed books, spreading plant knowledge beyond monastery walls. Nicholas Culpeper - part rebel, part bridge-builder - wrote in English rather than Latin, returning medicine to the hands of common people. He understood something essential: healing belongs to everyone, not just the credentialed few.

Yet here is what we must hold gently: one person's written record is not the whole story. It never is. Case and point, during the same timeframe that Nicholas Culpeper was being credited with rescuing the plight of herbal remedies for the layperson, his contemporary William Coles, delivered a scathing letter to Elias Ashmole, decrying Culpeper's disconnection from the plant world. He accused him of treading on plants and misleading his Countrymen with a false knowledge of simples and notions.

And still, it is Culpeper we acknowledge most notably in the modern world as a Renaissance father of herbal medicine. This information becomes valuable in understanding how knowledge of plant medicine has been shaped in the western world. One wonders, what our herbal legacy would be if Coles' work had been the leading work of the time?

For thousands of years before Hippocrates, before ink and parchment, European peoples lived in intimate conversation with their plant allies. Grandmothers passed remedies to daughters in kitchens and gardens. Healers read the land the way we read books. This knowledge traveled through hands, through song, through the body itself.

Most of it was never written down. Much of what was written was deliberately destroyed. What remains are fragments - Greek, Roman, Celtic texts - through which we glimpse an older, deeper knowing.

When we study European herbalism, we study what survived. Let us also honor what was lost - and trust that some of it still lives in the plants themselves, waiting to be remembered.

❧ Indigenous North American Traditions

Indigenous communities throughout North America maintained - and maintain - profound knowledge of locally available plants for food, medicine, shelter, and ceremony. This knowledge, developed over thousands of years of intimate observation and relationship with the land, represents sophisticated understanding that Western science is only beginning to recognize.

Colonization attempted to suppress much of this wisdom. Attempted. But plants are patient, and so are the peoples who love them. Many Indigenous communities have maintained and are now reclaiming their traditional plant knowledge, sharing it on their own terms and protecting it from exploitation.

As students of herbalism, our role here is not to extract or appropriate. It is to listen, when listening is offered. To support, when support is welcomed. And to tend our own ancestral lineages, whatever they may be, rather than reaching for what is not ours to take.

The Cultural Significance of Herbal Traditions

The cultural significance of herbal traditions runs deeper than their material benefits. Plants have played pivotal roles in health, spirituality, ceremony, and daily life across all cultures - not as tools, but as relatives.

Herbal traditions carry significant intergenerational wisdom. Knowledge thrives through oral histories, shared practices, and the preservation of ancestral teachings. Elders in various communities serve as custodians of this knowledge, imparting it to younger generations through apprenticeship and storytelling - the same way you are receiving it now, through a different kind of page.

These practices are repositories of cultural identity, connecting people to their ancestors, their land, and their way of understanding the world. When herbal knowledge is lost, an entire worldview can disappear with it. When it is preserved and passed on, something of the ancestors continues to live.

The incorporation of herbal traditions into modern integrative systems demonstrates their enduring relevance. Herbal remedies, once relegated to the margins of scientific inquiry, are now subjects of rigorous research validating what traditional practitioners have known for centuries. The plants were right all along. The grandmothers were right all along.

Modern Herbal Medicine

The advent of modern medicine in the 19th and 20th centuries brought significant transformations to herbal practice - both challenges and opportunities. While synthetic pharmaceuticals gained dominance in Western healthcare systems, herbal medicine never disappeared. It simply went underground, tended in kitchens and gardens, passed quietly from hand to hand.

Today, herbal medicine is experiencing renewed interest as individuals seek complementary and alternative approaches to health and wellness. The World Health Organization estimates that 80% of the global population relies primarily on traditional medicine, much of it plant-based. We in the industrialized West are the anomaly, not the norm.

The growing emphasis on personalized medicine, preventive care, and whole-systems approaches aligns beautifully with herbal medicine's strengths. Rather than viewing herbs and pharmaceuticals as adversaries, integrative approaches recognize that both have valuable roles to play - that the question is not "which is better" but "what does this person, in this moment, need?"

It's worth noting that many modern pharmaceuticals are derived from plants or synthesized versions of plant compounds - aspirin from willow bark, digoxin from foxglove, taxol from Pacific yew, artemisinin from sweet wormwood. The pharmaceutical industry knows the power of plants. It simply prefers to isolate, patent, and profit rather than honor the whole.

This underscores plants' chemical sophistication and therapeutic potential - potential we're still only beginning to understand through a scientific lens. The plants have always been medicine. We are just remembering how to see it.

Ethical Considerations in Modern Herbalism

As you cross the threshold into herbal practice, ethical considerations must guide your path. The relationship between humans and medicinal plants carries responsibilities - not as rules imposed from outside, but as the natural consequence of being in right relationship.

❧ Sustainability

Sustainability is critical as global demand for herbal remedies continues to rise. Overharvesting and habitat destruction threaten the availability of many medicinal species. Plants like American ginseng, goldenseal, and many orchids used in traditional medicine face serious population declines. Some may disappear entirely within our lifetimes if we do not change.

As an herbalist, you step into a lineage of responsibility. This means learning which plants are at risk before wildcrafting - before you ever put hand to stem. It means harvesting respectfully, never taking more than you need, and often taking less than you could. It means growing your own herbs whenever possible, so wild populations can recover. It means supporting companies that source herbs sustainably, even when that costs more. It means speaking up for plant conservation in a world that often forgets that plants are beings, not products.

You cannot be in relationship with plants while participating in their extinction. These two things cannot coexist.

❧ Safety

Safety is paramount in herbal practice. The assumption that "natural equals safe" is not only incorrect - it's dangerous. Plants are powerful medicine, and powerful medicine requires respect and knowledge. Hemlock is natural. Poison ivy is natural. Nature is not a synonym for harmless.

Challenges in herbal safety include the lack of standardization in many commercial products, potential interactions with pharmaceuticals, contamination or adulteration by unscrupulous suppliers, misidentification of plants by inexperienced harvesters, and inappropriate dosing by those who assume more is always better.

Your responsibility as a student and future practitioner is to study thoroughly before using or recommending any herb. To understand contraindications and interactions. To source herbs from reputable suppliers you have vetted. To consult with experienced practitioners when you are uncertain. To know the limits of your knowledge and when to refer to medical professionals. Humility is not weakness here - it is wisdom.

The plants deserve practitioners who take their power seriously. So do the people who come to you for help.

❧ Cultural Respect and Appropriation

Many medicinal plants are inseparable from the cultural and spiritual practices of the peoples who have stewarded them for generations. As you learn about herbs from various traditions, approach with humility and respect. You are a guest in someone else's ancestral home.

Cultural appropriation occurs when sacred practices are commercialized without permission, when traditional knowledge is patented by outsiders for profit, when plants are harvested without regard for Indigenous sovereignty, when cultural practices are trivialized, exoticized, or misrepresented. It is taking without relationship. Consuming without reciprocity.

Instead, practice cultural respect by learning the history and cultural context of the plants and practices you encounter. Support Indigenous and traditional practitioners directly when you can. Do not claim to practice traditions you haven't been initiated into - wearing the costume of someone else's lineage helps no one. Give credit to the cultural origins of knowledge. Understand that some knowledge is not meant to be shared outside its context, and honor those boundaries even when your curiosity pushes against them.

The deepest path is often to turn toward your own ancestors. What plant wisdom lives in your own lineage, waiting to be reclaimed?

❧ Reciprocity: The Foundation of Relationship

This brings us to perhaps the most important concept in this chapter: *reciprocity*.

Reciprocity means mutual exchange - giving as well as taking. In relationship with plants, this means we don't just harvest their medicine. We give something back. We complete the circle.

What can you offer in reciprocity?

To individual plants: careful, respectful harvesting that allows them to continue thriving. Spreading their seeds. Improving their habitat. Sitting with them in appreciation, offering your attention and presence. Water when they're dry. Companionship when they're alone.

To plant communities: protecting habitat from development and destruction. Removing invasive species that crowd out natives. Planting native species where they've been lost. Speaking up for conservation. Supporting organizations that protect wild places.

To the more-than-human world: living more lightly on the earth. Reducing consumption. Composting, recycling, regenerating. Teaching others to value and protect plants. Using your skills in service to something larger than yourself.

To human communities: sharing plant medicine with those who need it. Teaching others about plants. Preserving and passing on traditional knowledge with integrity. Supporting Indigenous sovereignty and traditional practitioners. Making medicine accessible, not exploitative.

Reciprocity transforms your relationship with plants from extraction to exchange. You are not taking from passive resources. You are in relationship with living beings who give to you, and to whom you give in return.

This is the foundation of ethical, sustainable, sacred herbalism. This is what makes it medicine and not just pharmacology.

Stepping Across

You've read about history, culture, ethics, reciprocity.

But none of this becomes real until you actually sit with a plant. Until you meet them on their own terms, as sovereign beings rather than ingredients or information.

This is your invitation: Go outside. Find a plant - any plant. You don't need to know its name yet. Names come later. Relationship comes first.

Just sit with it. Look at it - really look. Notice its leaves, its stems, its flowers or seeds if it has them. The way light moves through it. The way it holds itself in space. Smell it. Touch it gently, asking permission first.

Then ask: *What do you want me to know?*

And listen. Not with your ears, but with your whole being. What arises? What do you notice in your body? What images or feelings or knowings come through?

This is the beginning of relationship.

This is the threshold crossed.

Welcome.

Embodied Practice: The Communion of Breath

Before you close this chapter, I want to offer you a practice - something to move this knowledge from your mind into your body, from concept into lived experience. This is the kind of work we do together in class, and it belongs here too.

This practice requires nothing but yourself and a few quiet minutes. You can do it indoors or outside. You can do it with a houseplant on your windowsill or a tree you pass on your daily walk. You can return to it again and again throughout this course - it will deepen each time.

Read through the entire practice first. Then set down the book, close your eyes, and let your body lead.

❧ Preparing the Container

Find a comfortable position - seated or standing, whatever allows you to be both relaxed and alert. If you're with a plant, position yourself so you can see it easily, or touch it if that feels right.

Close your eyes. Take three slow breaths, letting each exhale be a little longer than the inhale. With each breath out, let your shoulders soften. Let your jaw release. Let your belly be soft.

Feel the weight of your body. Feel where you make contact with the earth - through your feet, your seat, whatever touches ground. Let yourself be held.

Now bring your attention to the simple fact of your breathing. You breathe in. You breathe out. This is happening without your effort, without your control. Your body knows how to do this. It has been doing it since the moment you were born.

❧ The Ancient Exchange

Now consider this: with every breath you take, you are in conversation with the plant world.

You breathe in oxygen - the breath plants have exhaled. You breathe out carbon dioxide - the breath plants will inhale. This is not metaphor. This is not poetry. This is the literal, biological truth of your existence. Your lungs and a leaf are two halves of the same breathing.

Let this land in your body. Feel it. You are breathing with the green world right now. You always have been.

As you inhale, imagine you are receiving a gift from the plants - their out-breath becoming your in-breath. Let yourself feel gratitude for this. Let yourself feel the intimacy of it. They are keeping you alive with every breath.

As you exhale, imagine you are offering a gift in return - your out-breath becoming their in-breath. You are feeding them. You are part of their survival too. This is reciprocity at its most fundamental.

Breathe with this awareness for several minutes. There is nothing to achieve. Just breathe, and know that you are in relationship.

❧ Deepening the Connection

If you are with a specific plant - a houseplant, a garden herb, a tree outside your window - open your eyes softly now. Let your gaze rest on the plant without staring, without analyzing. Just be with it the way you might be with a friend in comfortable silence.

Notice what you notice. The color of the leaves - not "green" but *this* green, this particular shade that belongs to this plant. The texture. The way it holds itself - upright or trailing, compact or sprawling. The way light touches it.

What is your body doing as you look? What do you feel in your chest, your belly, your hands? These sensations are information. They are part of how plants speak to us.

Now, silently or aloud, offer a greeting. It might be as simple as "Hello" or "I see you" or "Thank you for being here." Notice if anything shifts - in you or in the space between you and the plant.

If you feel moved to, ask the plant: *What would you have me know?*

Then simply wait. Listen with your whole body. The answer may come as words, or as an image, or as a feeling, or as a sudden knowing. It may come now or later - in a dream, in a flash of insight while washing dishes. It may come as silence, which is also an answer.

There is no wrong way to do this. There is no way to fail. You are simply practicing presence. You are simply saying, with your attention: *I am here. I am willing. I am listening.*

❧ Closing the Practice

When you feel complete - and you will know - offer thanks. Thank the plant for its presence, for its breath, for whatever it has shared with you. Thank your own body for being the vessel of this experience.

Take three more slow breaths. With each exhale, let yourself return gently to ordinary awareness - but carrying something with you. Something has shifted. Something has begun.

Open your eyes fully. Feel your feet on the ground. Wiggle your fingers. You are here, in your body, in this moment.

You have just crossed the threshold.

❧ Integration

After this practice, you may want to write. Not an analysis - just whatever wants to come through. Stream of consciousness, images, fragments, questions. Your journal is a place to catch what the practice stirred before it fades.

Some questions to sit with:
What did I notice in my body during the practice?

Was there a moment when I felt something shift?
What surprised me?
If the plant communicated something, what was it? (Even if I'm not sure, even if it seems like I'm making it up - what came?)
What do I want to remember from this experience?

This practice is yours now. Return to it whenever you need to remember why you're here, what this path is really about. Return to it when the study feels heavy or the information overwhelming. The plants are always breathing. The conversation is always available. You just have to show up.

Recommended Further Reading

- *Braiding Sweetgrass* by Robin Wall Kimmerer - on reciprocity and Indigenous plant wisdom
- *Sacred Plant Medicine* by Stephen Harrod Buhner
- *The Lost Language of Plants* by Stephen Harrod Buhner
- *Medical Herbalism* by David Hoffmann - for clinical depth
- A field guide to medicinal plants in your bioregion - the plants in your place, waiting to meet you

Reflection Questions

1. What brought you to the study of herbal medicine? Not the practical reason - the deeper pull. What is it you're really seeking?

2. What does reciprocity mean to you? How might you practice it - not as concept, but as daily action?

3. Which herbal tradition(s) are you drawn to learn more about, and why? What do you sense they might offer you?

4. What ethical questions or concerns arise for you as you begin this path? What do you want to be careful about?

. . .

5. What did the plant you sat with teach you? What did you learn that you couldn't have learned from a book?

Welcome to the journey. The plants are waiting.

Chapter 2
Learning to Listen
Developing Plant Sensitivity & Energetic Awareness

You've crossed the threshold. You've sat with a plant and begun to build relationship. You've felt the ancient exchange of breath moving between your lungs and the green world.

Now we go deeper.

This chapter is about learning to listen more carefully - to sense what the plants are showing you through their taste, their temperature, their qualities. It's about developing the kind of sensory intelligence that allows you to know a plant not just by name, but by how it moves through your body. How it makes you *feel*.

We call this way of knowing *energetics* - an ancient approach to understanding how plants affect us, based not on laboratory analysis but on direct sensory experience. You will learn to taste, to feel, to observe with all your senses. You will learn to trust what your body tells you.

This chapter provides the conceptual framework. But the real learning happens when you put plants in your mouth, feel them move through your system, and document what *you* experience. No book can give you that. Only the plants can. Only your own body can.

What Are Energetics?

Energetics - sometimes called herbal energetics or plant energetics - is a traditional way of describing the qualities of medicinal plants. It emphasizes the understanding that plants possess specific properties that can affect our physical and emotional well-being in predictable ways.

Think of it this way: if you've ever eaten a raw jalapeño, you didn't need a chemistry textbook to tell you it was heating. Your mouth knew. Your forehead knew, as sweat began to bead. Your whole body registered *hot*. That direct knowing - that immediate, embodied understanding of a plant's nature - is the foundation of energetics.

Understanding these energetic properties allows herbalists to match plants to people based on their constitutional needs and current conditions - not just their symptoms. Two people with the same headache might need completely different herbs, because the *pattern* underneath the headache is different. One runs hot; one runs cold. One is tense; one is depleted. Energetics helps us see these patterns.

This approach has deep roots. Nicholas Culpeper, the 17th-century English herbalist who brought medicine back to common people, wrote extensively about the importance of understanding plant energetics. His approach drew from ancient Greek and medieval humoralism - the understanding that imbalances in bodily fluids could be corrected through herbs with specific qualities. Hot herbs for cold conditions. Dry herbs for damp conditions. Balance restored through opposites.

We don't use humoral theory exactly as it was practiced historically. But the core principle remains as true as it ever was: plants have qualities that can help rebalance the body. And we can learn to perceive those qualities directly, through our own senses, the same way humans have for thousands of years.

The Primary Energetic Qualities

There are various ways to categorize a plant's energetics, but they often involve pairs of opposing qualities. These are not abstract categories - they are descriptions of what you will actually *feel* when you work with plants. Let's explore the most fundamental.

❧ Temperature: The Spectrum of Hot to Cold

This is perhaps the most important energetic quality - and the one your body will recognize most readily. It's not about the physical temperature of the plant, but about how it affects *your* temperature when you take it.

Hot and warming herbs - like ginger, cayenne, cinnamon, and black pepper - create heat in the body. They stimulate circulation, increase metabolism, disperse congestion and stagnation. When you eat fresh ginger, you feel it: the warmth building in your mouth, spreading through your chest, perhaps even making you sweat. That's the plant's heating nature, experienced directly.

Cool and cooling herbs - like peppermint, violet, chickweed, and lemon balm - do the opposite. They reduce excess heat, calm inflammation, soothe irritated tissues, help break fevers. When you chew a fresh peppermint leaf, you feel that immediate cooling, that sense of opening and clearing. That's the plant's cooling nature.

When do we reach for warming herbs? When there's coldness in the body - poor circulation, always feeling chilled, things feeling stuck or blocked or heavy. When digestion is slow and sluggish. When dampness sits heavy with cold underneath it.

When do we reach for cooling herbs? When there's excess heat - fever, hot flashes, burning sensations, inflammation showing as redness and swelling and irritation. When tissues are dry and parched and thirsty.

Your own body already knows how to recognize temperature. You just need to pay attention.

❧ Moisture: The Spectrum of Dry to Moist

This quality describes how herbs affect the body's fluids and tissues - whether they dry things out or add moisture back in.

Drying herbs reduce excess moisture, dry up secretions, and have astringent properties that tighten and tone tissues. Yarrow, oak bark, sage, witch hazel - these plants pull things together, reduce what's leaking or overflowing. You can often recognize drying herbs by their astringent taste, that puckering sensation that draws the tissues of your mouth together.

Moistening herbs - the demulcents - do the opposite. They add moisture to dry tissues, soothe and protect mucous membranes, coat and calm irritation. Marshmallow root, slippery elm, licorice root, violet leaf - these plants bring the quality of water, of nourishment, of soothing presence. When you drink a cold infusion of marshmallow root, you feel that slippery, coating quality immediately. That's the plant's moistening nature.

Reach for drying herbs when there's excess moisture - a runny nose that won't stop, watery diarrhea, excessive sweating, lax and boggy tissues, edema and water retention. Reach for moistening herbs when there's dryness - dry skin, dry cough, constipation, irritated and inflamed mucous membranes, thirst that doesn't seem to quench.

Energy: The Spectrum of Stimulating to Relaxing

This describes the herb's effect on the nervous system and overall vital energy - whether it revs things up or settles them down.

Stimulating herbs increase alertness, improve circulation, enhance metabolism, and move stagnation. Rosemary, ginger, coffee, green tea - these plants wake things up, get things moving, bring energy and clarity. Sometimes we need this. Sometimes the system has become too slow, too stuck, too sleepy.

Relaxing herbs calm the nervous system, ease tension, promote sleep, and reduce spasm. Chamomile, lemon balm, passionflower, valerian - these plants settle things down, release what's gripped, invite rest. And sometimes *this* is what we need - to be unwound, unheld, allowed to soften.

Notice that these are not value judgments. Stimulating is not better than relaxing, or vice versa. They are different medicines for different moments, different constitutions, different needs.

Understanding Your Own Constitution

To match plants to people, you first need to understand your own constitutional tendencies. These are the patterns your body naturally inclines toward when it falls out of balance - your particular way of going off-center.

Some of us run hot. We tend toward warmth, heat easily, may experience inflammation frequently. Red complexion, perhaps a quick temper. We prefer cool weather and cooling foods, and we generally benefit from cooling herbs.

Some of us run cold. Always feeling chilled, especially in the hands and feet. Slow metabolism, low energy. Pale complexion, perhaps soft-spoken. We crave warmth and generally benefit from warming herbs.

Some of us tend toward dryness - dry skin, dry hair, dry lips. Prone to constipation. Often thin in build. We benefit from moistening, nourishing herbs.

Some of us tend toward dampness - retaining water easily, producing excess mucus, feeling heavy and sluggish. We benefit from drying, moving herbs.

Some of us hold tension - in our muscles, in our minds. Anxious, stressed, wound tight, difficulty letting go. We benefit from relaxing, calming herbs.

Most of us are combinations of these qualities. You might be cold and damp, or hot and dry, or tense and cold. Understanding your particular pattern helps you choose herbs that bring you back toward balance - not someone else's balance, but your own.

What is your tendency? You probably already know, if you listen to what your body has been telling you all along.

Meeting Specific Plants Through Their Energetics

Let's make these concepts concrete by exploring several plants you can actually meet, taste, and experience for yourself. These are not just profiles to memorize - they are invitations to relationship.

Peppermint (Mentha x piperita)

Energetics: Cooling, drying, dispersing

Peppermint is widely recognized for its ability to ease digestive discomfort - bloating, gas, nausea. Its antispasmodic and carminative qualities make it invaluable for soothing gastrointestinal distress. But peppermint is more than a stomach remedy. It has an invigorating, clarifying quality that clears the head and opens the breath.

Energetically, peppermint is cooling and dispersing - it clears heat, invigorates the senses, and moves stagnation outward. This makes it particularly suited for conditions characterized by heat or congestion in the body. Hot headaches. Digestive heat and tension. Mental fogginess that needs clearing. Fevers that need to break.

When might you *not* reach for peppermint? When someone is already very cold - peppermint will make that worse. When there's GERD, because peppermint can relax the lower esophageal sphincter. When conditions are very dry - peppermint's drying quality can worsen dryness.

Your experience: Chew a fresh peppermint leaf, or drink unsweetened peppermint tea. Notice the immediate cooling sensation. Notice how it opens your breathing, how clarity comes to your mind. Feel for any tingling, any dispersing quality. *This* is what "cooling and dispersing" actually means - not as concept, but as felt reality.

Ginger (Zingiber officinale)

Energetics: Hot, drying, stimulating, dispersing

Ginger is one of our most important warming herbs - a rhizome that has been used across cultures for thousands of years for digestive support, nausea relief, pain reduction, and to kindle the digestive fire. It is known for its anti-inflammatory and antioxidant properties, but these clinical terms don't quite capture what ginger *does*.

Energetically, ginger is one of our hottest herbs. It creates heat, stimulates circulation, disperses stagnation, and moves energy that has become stuck. This makes it invaluable for cold conditions - poor circulation, feeling chilled, slow digestion, no appetite. Ginger can also help move congested mucus and is often added to formulas to activate and harmonize other herbs.

When might you *not* reach for ginger? When someone is already running hot - fever, hot flashes, active inflammation. Use with caution during bleeding, as ginger moves blood. Be mindful with high doses alongside blood-thinning medications.

Your experience: Chew a thin slice of fresh raw ginger. Feel the immediate heat building. Notice how it spreads through your mouth and throat, perhaps down into your belly. Notice the increased saliva, the warmth that might spread to your whole body. Feel the dispersing, almost explosive quality. If you start to sweat, that's ginger doing what ginger does. *This* is what "hot and dispersing" feels like in your own body.

Marshmallow Root (Althaea officinalis)

Energetics: Cooling, moistening, soothing

Marshmallow root has been used for centuries for its remarkable soothing and demulcent properties. It contains mucilage - a gelatinous substance that coats and protects mucous membranes, offering relief for sore throats, digestive irritation, and urinary tract discomfort. Where ginger is fire, marshmallow is water - cool, gentle, nourishing.

Energetically, marshmallow root is cooling and deeply moistening, making it especially suited for conditions characterized by dryness and heat. Dry coughs, sore throats, digestive inflammation, urinary irritation, dry and irritated skin - anywhere tissues are parched and inflamed, marshmallow brings relief.

Your experience: Make a cold infusion of marshmallow root - place one tablespoon of dried root in a cup of cold water, let it steep overnight, then strain. Drink it slowly. Notice the slippery, coating sensation as it moves through your mouth and throat. Feel how it soothes, how it calms. Notice the cooling quality, how long the soothing effect lasts. *This* is what "demulcent" and "moistening" mean - not as vocabulary to memorize, but as medicine you can feel.

Calendula (Calendula officinalis)

Energetics: Warming, drying, moving

Calendula - sometimes called pot marigold - is renowned for its wound-healing and anti-inflammatory properties. Applied topically in salves, creams, or infused oils, it supports the healing of cuts, burns, rashes, and insect bites. It stimulates collagen production and encourages tissue regeneration. Those bright orange and yellow flowers carry powerful medicine.

Energetically, calendula is warming and drying, making it particularly effective for conditions associated with dampness or stagnation. Its warming nature supports circulation and stimulates the movement of fluids, helping to reduce swelling and resolve stuck conditions. It has an affinity for the lymphatic system - those quiet rivers that carry waste and immune cells through the body.

Reach for calendula when wounds need healing, when lymph feels stagnant, when damp skin conditions persist, when inflammation carries a quality of dampness beneath it.

The Six Tastes and Their Wisdom

Traditional systems around the world recognized that taste itself carries information about a plant's properties. Your tongue is not just for pleasure - it's a diagnostic tool, a way of reading a plant's nature before it even reaches your stomach.

Bitter **plants** - dandelion, gentian, goldenseal - tend to be cooling and drying. They stimulate digestion, drain dampness, and wake up sluggish organs. That challenging taste you might want to spit out? It's medicine for a system that has become too comfortable, too slow.

Sweet **plants** - licorice, marshmallow, oats - tend to be neutral to warm and moistening. They nourish, build, and tonify. Sweetness (not sugar, but the true sweet taste of nourishing plants) is the taste of sustenance, of restoration.

Pungent or spicy **plants** - ginger, cayenne, garlic - tend to be warming and drying. They disperse, move, and stimulate. When you feel that heat spread through your body, that's the pungent taste doing its work of breaking up stagnation.

Sour **plants** - hawthorn berry, rose hips, lemon - tend to be cooling and drying. They have an astringent, contracting quality that preserves fluids while tightening what has become too lax.

Salty **plants** - bladderwrack, kelp, sea vegetables - tend to be cooling to neutral and moistening. They soften hardness, open what has become closed, and bring the mineral richness of the sea.

Astringent **plants** - witch hazel, oak bark, raspberry leaf - tend to be cooling and drying. They tighten, tone, and stop leakage. That puckering sensation in your mouth? It's the plant showing you how it will work in your body.

When you taste a plant mindfully, you are receiving a message about its nature. *Trust your tongue.*

Developing Your Sensory Intelligence

Reading about energetics is useful. But the real learning - the learning that lives in your body and cannot be forgotten - comes from direct sensory experience. Here's how to cultivate this skill.

For each herb you study, begin by observing before tasting. Look at the plant or dried herb with fresh eyes, as if you've never seen it before. Notice color, texture, shape. Smell it - what arises? What does it remind you of? What do you feel in your body just from the smell?

Then taste mindfully. Chew a small amount of dried herb or fresh plant (if it's safe and you've identified it correctly). Let it sit on your tongue. Notice the immediate sensations - is it hot or cool? Bitter, sweet, sour, salty, pungent, astringent? How does it make your mouth feel - dry, wet, tingly, numb?

Then track the effects as they unfold. What happens in the next few minutes? Do you feel warmth spreading, or cooling? Moistening, or drying? Does your mind become more alert or more calm? What happens in your belly, your chest, your limbs?

Document everything. Write down what you noticed, what surprised you, what you're not sure about. This becomes *your* materia medica - your personal record of relationship with plants. Your direct experience is as valid as anything in any book. More valid, actually, because it's yours.

Building Your Personal Materia Medica

A materia medica is a collection of knowledge about medicinal plants - their properties, uses, preparations. Traditionally, these were compiled by master herbalists over lifetimes of practice. You are beginning to build your own.

For each plant you come to know, gather the practical information: common and Latin names, plant family, parts used. Note the energetics - temperature, moisture, taste, and most importantly, your own direct experience of what the plant does in your body.

Document the actions - what does this plant do? Is it anti-inflammatory, digestive, nervine, immune-supporting? Note the traditional uses - what conditions has it been used for through history? Record preparation methods and dosage ranges. And be honest about contraindications - who should not use this herb, and what might it interact with?

But here is what I want you to include that most materia medicas leave out: your relationship with this plant. How does it make you feel? When do you reach for it? What has it taught you? What do you notice about the quality of its presence? These are not soft additions - they are the heart of the matter.

Your materia medica will grow throughout your life. Some entries will be detailed; some will be sketches. Some plants will become intimate friends; others will remain acquaintances. There's no wrong way to do this. You are building a record of relationship, written in the language of your own experience.

The Principle of Opposites - And Its Limits

A fundamental principle in energetic herbalism: opposite energetics tend to balance each other. Cold conditions need warming herbs. Hot conditions need cooling herbs. Dry conditions need moistening herbs. Damp conditions need drying herbs. Tense conditions need relaxing herbs. Lax conditions need toning herbs.

This is a useful starting principle. But don't hold it too rigidly.

Sometimes the body is asking for something more nuanced than simple opposites. Sometimes you need to work *with* a condition rather than against it. Sometimes what looks like excess is actually deficiency in disguise. A skilled herbalist learns when to use opposites and when to use supportive herbs that work alongside what's happening.

This discernment comes with practice, observation, and humility. You will make mistakes. You will learn from them. The plants are patient teachers.

Practicing Energetic Thinking

Let's practice applying this framework to real situations. These are not prescriptions - they are invitations to think energetically, to see patterns rather than just symptoms.

Imagine someone who feels cold all the time, with poor circulation and pale complexion, slow digestion and low energy. What pattern do you see? Cold, perhaps with some dampness if there's also sluggishness. What might help? Warming herbs like ginger, cinnamon, cayenne - perhaps warming tonics like astragalus if the cold comes from deep depletion.

Now imagine someone experiencing hot flashes, irritability, red face, burning digestion, and restlessness. What pattern? Excess heat. What might help? Cooling herbs like peppermint, violet, lemon balm - cooling nervines like skullcap if the heat is tangled with tension.

Someone with a dry cough, dry skin, constant thirst, and constipation? Dryness, possibly with heat. Moistening demulcents like marshmallow root, slippery elm - cooling moisteners like violet if heat is present.

Someone with excess mucus, watery diarrhea, feeling heavy and sluggish? Dampness, possibly with cold. Drying herbs like yarrow, sage - warming drying herbs if cold is also present.

Do you see how this works? You're reading the person, not just the symptom. You're matching plant qualities to human needs. This is the art of energetic herbalism.

Moving Forward

You now have a framework for understanding plant energetics. But remember: this is a map, not the territory. The map is useful. The territory is where you actually live.

The real learning happens when you taste herbs mindfully, when you document your own experiences, when you observe how plants affect *you* specifically. When you build relationships with plants over time. When you stay curious and humble.

Your senses are your teachers. The plants themselves are your teachers. Books - including this one - are guides. But experience is the real education. There is no substitute for putting a plant in your mouth and paying attention.

Embodied Practice: The Tasting Meditation

This practice is the heart of energetic herbalism - meeting a plant through your senses, letting your body be the teacher. You will need a single herb to taste. Choose something accessible and safe: dried peppermint, fresh ginger, chamomile flowers, a sprig of rosemary from the garden. What matters is not which herb you choose, but *how* you meet it.

Set aside twenty to thirty minutes when you won't be interrupted. Have your journal nearby. Read through the entire practice first, then set down the book and let your senses lead.

Arriving

Begin by settling into your body. Close your eyes. Take several slow breaths, letting each exhale carry away distraction and hurry. Feel your feet on the floor, your seat on the chair, your weight held by the earth.

Before you engage with the plant, take a moment to notice your baseline. How does your body feel right now, before you've taken anything? Notice your mouth - is it dry or moist? Notice your belly - calm, tense, warm, cool? Notice your energy - alert, tired, agitated, peaceful? Notice your temperature - are you running warm today, or cool?

This is your starting point. You need to know where you began to recognize where the plant takes you.

Meeting With the Eyes

Open your eyes and pick up the herb. Look at it as if you've never seen it before - because in this way, with this attention, you haven't.

What do you notice about its form? The color - not just "green" or "brown" but the specific shade, the variations. The texture - rough or smooth, hairy or glossy, thick or delicate. The shape - how the leaves are arranged, how it holds itself, what geometry it has chosen.

What does looking at this plant evoke in you? Any emotions, memories, associations? Any sense of its character, its personality? These impressions are information.

Meeting With the Nose

Bring the herb to your nose. Breathe in slowly through your nostrils. What arrives?

Don't rush to name it. Just receive the scent. Is it sharp or soft? Heavy or light? Does it rise quickly and fade, or linger? Does it remind you of anything?

Notice what happens in your body as you smell the plant. Some herbs will make you salivate. Some will make you want to breathe more deeply. Some might make you pull back. Your body is already reading the plant's nature.

Smell is one of our oldest senses, wired directly to memory and emotion. Trust what it tells you.

❧ Meeting With the Mouth

Now the central practice: tasting.

Place a small amount of the herb in your mouth. If it's dried herb, just a pinch. If it's fresh ginger, a thin slice. If it's a flower, a single blossom. You don't need much - this is about attention, not quantity.

Let it sit on your tongue for a moment before you begin to chew. What do you taste immediately? Bitter, sweet, sour, salty, pungent? Perhaps a combination? Perhaps something you can't quite name?

Now begin to chew slowly. Notice how the taste changes as you break down the plant material. Notice what happens in your mouth - is it becoming more moist or more dry? Is there a warming sensation, or cooling? Tingling? Numbness? Puckering?

Let the herb stay in your mouth longer than you normally would. This is not eating - it's listening. Your mouth is gathering information about who this plant is.

❧ Meeting With the Whole Body

Swallow when you're ready. And now pay attention to what happens next.

Track the sensations as the herb moves down your throat. Does the taste linger? Does the cooling or warming quality persist? What do you notice in your esophagus, your chest, your belly?

Over the next several minutes, widen your attention to your whole body. Has your energy shifted - are you more alert, more calm, more something else? Has your temperature changed? Do you notice anything in your head, your sinuses, your limbs? Any emotions arising?

This is the plant teaching you its nature. Not through words, but through what it does in your body. This is knowledge you cannot get from any book.

❧ Recording

After sitting with the experience for five to ten minutes, open your journal and write.

Don't worry about getting it "right." Just record what you noticed, as simply and honestly as you can. Include the surprises, the subtleties, the things you're not sure about. Note the date, the plant you tasted, and anything relevant about your state beforehand.

Some prompts to guide your writing:
What taste(s) did I notice? How did they change over time?
Did the plant feel warming, cooling, or neutral? Where did I feel this in my body?
Did it feel moistening, drying, or neutral?
Did it feel stimulating, relaxing, or neutral?
What surprised me?
If I had to describe this plant's personality in a few words, what would I say?

Closing

When your writing feels complete, take a moment to thank the plant. Not because you have to, but because gratitude completes the exchange. You received something - information, medicine, relationship. Let your thanks be the gift you offer in return.

Take three slow breaths. Feel your feet on the ground. You have just added to your personal materia medica - not with someone else's words, but with your own direct experience.

Return to this practice regularly. Taste one herb, then another. Taste the same herb on different days, in different seasons, in different states of health. Your materia medica will grow, and so will your capacity to listen.

Recommended Practices

- *Daily herb tasting:* Choose one herb each day. Taste it mindfully. Document your experience. Over weeks, this builds a rich, personal materia medica.
- *Temperature awareness:* Throughout each day, notice - do you tend hot or cold? When? What seems to influence it? Begin to know your patterns.
- *Moisture awareness:* Pay attention to your moisture level - skin, mouth, digestion. What do you notice? What does your body seem to need?
- *Energetic journaling:* Keep notes on how different herbs affect you specifically. What works for you may differ from what works for someone else. You are learning your own constitution.
- *Seasonal observations:* Notice how the seasons affect your energetic balance. Does winter make you more cold and dry? Does summer bring heat? Let the seasons teach you about yourself.

Reflection Questions

1. What is your constitutional tendency? Hot or cold? Dry or damp? Tense or relaxed? How do you know?

2. How did it feel to taste herbs mindfully, with full attention? What surprised you?

3. Which energetic quality do you think you need most support with right now? Why?

4. How does this framework of energetics change the way you think about plants - and about yourself?

5. What questions remain for you about energetics? What do you want to explore further?

Further Reading

- *The Energetics of Western Herbs* by Peter Holmes - comprehensive and deep
- *The Practice of Traditional Western Herbalism* by Matthew Wood - intuitive and accessible
- *Planetary Herbology* by Michael Tierra - bridging traditions
- Your own growing materia medica - built from direct experience, the most important text you'll ever read.

Your direct experience is the primary text.
Everything else is commentary.
Trust your senses. Build relationships. The plants are waiting to teach you.

Chapter 3
Learning Their Language
The Alchemy of Extraction & Preparation

The Language of Preparation

You've learned to listen to plants, to sense their energetics through your own body. You've begun to build relationships through breath and attention and taste.

Now you learn to speak back.

Each method of preparation - tea, tincture, salve, syrup - is a different kind of conversation with the plant. Some methods coax out what dissolves in water; others call forth what releases only into alcohol or oil. Some approaches are gentle, a soft invitation; others are more insistent, drawing out constituents through heat or time or pressure. Some preparations must be used immediately, fresh and alive; others can wait years on a shelf, holding their potency in amber glass.

Learning these methods is learning how to ask plants for different gifts. It is learning the grammar of transformation - how water becomes tea, how oil becomes salve, how alcohol becomes tincture. It is alchemy in the truest sense: the art of drawing essence from matter, of making medicine from plant.

This chapter provides the foundational knowledge. But the real learning happens in your kitchen, with your hands in herbs, making medicine the way humans have made it for thousands of years. The techniques matter. But so does the presence you bring, the attention, the care. Plants know when they're being handled with love.

Choosing Your Method

Different methods of preparation suit different plants, different needs, different moments. Before you begin making medicine, you ask yourself several questions.

What part of the plant are you working with? Delicate flowers and soft leaves yield their gifts easily - a simple infusion is often enough. Tough roots and dense bark need more persuasion - a decoction that simmers, drawing out what doesn't release quickly. Tinctures work for either, given time. External preparations - salves, oils, poultices - speak directly to the skin.

What constituents are you trying to extract? Some plant compounds dissolve readily in water - tannins, mucilage, many minerals. Tea will draw these out. Other constituents - resins, certain alkaloids, volatile oils - prefer alcohol or oil as their medium. Knowing what you're after helps you choose the right solvent for the conversation.

How will the medicine be used? Internal preparations - teas, tinctures, syrups - are taken by mouth, moving through the digestive system into the blood. External preparations - salves, oils, poultices, compresses, baths - are applied to the skin, working locally or absorbing more slowly. Some situations call for quick action; others for slow, steady support over time.

Who will be using this medicine? A child needs gentler preparations - mild teas, syrups sweetened with honey, glycerites instead of alcohol tinctures. Someone recovering from addiction needs alternatives to alcohol-based medicines. Someone with a busy life might need the convenience of a tincture bottle in a purse; someone with more spacious mornings might prefer the ritual of brewing tea.

How long must the medicine last? Fresh tea should be drunk within a day. Syrups last months in the refrigerator. Tinctures can hold their potency for years. If you're making medicine for an acute situation, freshness matters more than preservation. If you're stocking your apothecary for the long haul, shelf life becomes a consideration.

There is no single right way to prepare any herb. Each method reveals different aspects of the plant's medicine. As you learn, you'll develop intuition about which preparation serves which situation - and which preparation calls to you for this plant, this moment, this need.

Water Preparations: The Simplest Alchemy

Water is the first solvent, the most ancient medium for extracting plant medicine. When you steep herbs in water, you're participating in a ritual older than recorded history - the transformation of plant matter into drinkable healing.

❧ Infusion: The Gentle Invitation

An infusion - what most people simply call tea - is a gentle method of drawing medicine from delicate plant materials: leaves, flowers, soft stems. The process is simple, almost domestic, but don't let that fool you. There is deep magic in a cup of properly made herbal tea.

The basic method: Measure approximately one tablespoon of dried herbs - or two tablespoons of fresh - per cup of water. Place the herbs in a teapot, a French press, or a simple mason jar. Pour boiling water over the herbs and cover immediately. This covering matters more than many people realize - it keeps the volatile oils from escaping into the air, where they would carry away part of the plant's medicine. Let the herbs steep for ten to fifteen minutes, longer than you would for a culinary tea. You're making medicine, not a mild beverage. Strain and drink while warm.

For mineral-rich herbs - nettles, oatstraw, red clover, horsetail - a long-steep infusion draws out the deep nourishment. Use four to six tablespoons of dried herb per quart of water and let it steep for four to eight hours, even overnight. The resulting brew will be darker, stronger, more earthy. This is where the minerals live - the calcium, the magnesium, the iron that builds blood and bone.

Infusions work beautifully for leaves like peppermint, lemon balm, nettles, and raspberry leaf. For flowers like chamomile, elderflower, lavender, and rose. For delicate aromatics that would lose their essential nature under prolonged heat. When you smell that fragrance rising from your cup, you're sensing the volatile oils that a long decoction would have driven off.

Drink your infusion within twenty-four hours. Unlike alcohol preparations, tea doesn't preserve well - it's living medicine that begins to change almost as soon as it's made. You can make it in larger batches and refrigerate, but know that you're drinking something closer to fresh than preserved. This is part of its gift: immediacy, presence, the medicine of now.

Decoction: The Patient Extraction

A decoction is for the tougher plant materials - the roots, barks, seeds, and stems that don't yield their medicine easily. Where an infusion is a gentle invitation, a decoction is a more sustained conversation, using time and heat to draw out what would otherwise remain locked inside.

The method: Place one tablespoon of dried root, bark, or seeds per cup of water in a pot. Use cold water to start - this gives the tough material time to begin softening before the heat intensifies. Bring to a boil, then reduce to a gentle simmer. Cover the pot and let it simmer for fifteen to thirty minutes, sometimes longer for very dense materials. Some roots want forty-five minutes. Medicinal mushrooms like reishi and chaga ask for two to four hours of patient simmering. The medicine is in no hurry.

Decoctions are how we work with roots like burdock, dandelion, ginger, licorice, and astragalus. With barks like cinnamon, cramp bark, and willow. With seeds like fennel and fenugreek. If you're working with tough material and wondering whether to infuse or decoct, decoct. The extra heat and time ensure that you're actually getting the medicine out.

A practical note: when you're working with a formula that includes both roots and leaves, decoct the roots first, then remove from heat and add the leaves to steep in the cooling liquid. This way each plant part receives the treatment it needs - the roots get their long simmer, the leaves get their gentle infusion, and nothing is overdone or underdone.

Cutting or grinding tough roots before decocting helps the water reach more surface area, extracting more efficiently. Your decoction can be refrigerated and gently reheated. Some people make a large batch at the beginning of the week and warm cups as needed - a practical approach when life is busy, but medicine is still required.

Alcohol Preparations: The Deep Extraction

Alcohol has been used to extract plant medicine for centuries, and for good reason. It pulls out both water-soluble and alcohol-soluble constituents, reaching compounds that water alone cannot touch. It preserves for years. It concentrates the medicine into small, portable doses. A tincture is patience transformed into power.

❧ Tinctures: Concentrated Conversations

A tincture is an alcohol-based preparation - herbs macerated in alcohol until the liquid has drawn out their medicine. The result is concentrated, long-lasting, and convenient. A small bottle of tincture can hold months of medicine, ready when you need it.

The folk method is forgiving and accessible, perfect for learning. First, choose your alcohol. Vodka at 40% (80 proof) works well for most dried herbs - it's neutral in flavor and strong enough to extract and preserve. Brandy is traditional, adding its own warmth to the medicine. Grain alcohol at 95% (190 proof) is necessary for resins and very tough materials, though you'll dilute it for most uses. Some people use apple cider vinegar for an alcohol-free extraction, though technically this creates an acetum rather than a true tincture.

Prepare your herbs by chopping or grinding them to increase surface area. Most herbs are tinctured dry, but some - lemon balm, St. John's wort, fresh echinacea root - are best tinctured fresh, when certain constituents are at their peak. Fill your jar one-third to one-half full with dried herbs (more if they're light and fluffy), or three-quarters full with fresh herbs (they'll compact as they release moisture).

Pour alcohol over the herbs until they're completely submerged with at least two inches of liquid above them. This matters - any plant material exposed to air will mold. Press down floating herbs. Make sure everything is covered.

Label your jar immediately and thoroughly: the herb name, the date, the type of alcohol, any notes. You will forget if you don't write it down. Every herbalist learns this lesson the hard way, staring at an unlabeled jar of mysterious brown liquid, trying to remember what they made six months ago.

Store your jar in a cool, dark place. Shake it daily, or at least every few days - this keeps the extraction moving, prevents settling, and is also a way of tending the medicine, remembering it, staying in relationship with the transformation happening inside. Let it macerate for four to six weeks. In a pinch, two weeks will do, but longer is stronger.

When the time has come, strain through a fine mesh strainer lined with cheesecloth. Squeeze the herbs to extract every drop of medicine - don't be shy about this. Compost the spent plant material. Store your tincture in dark amber bottles, labeled again with herb name and date. Properly stored, tinctures remain potent for three to five years, sometimes longer.

Standard dosing is thirty to sixty drops - about one to two milliliters - taken two to four times daily, though this varies by herb and situation. Tinctures can be dropped directly under the tongue for fastest absorption, or added to water, juice, or tea. Some people add their dose to hot water and let the alcohol evaporate slightly before drinking, which can make strong tinctures more palatable.

A note about who shouldn't use tinctures: anyone in recovery from alcohol addiction deserves medicine that doesn't threaten their sobriety. For them, choose teas, glycerites, or other preparations. Children need tinctures heavily diluted or avoided entirely - syrups and glycerites serve them better. Those who avoid alcohol for religious or personal reasons have every right to their convictions. There are always other ways to access a plant's medicine.

❧ Glycerites: The Sweet Alternative

Glycerites follow the same basic method as tinctures, but substitute vegetable glycerin for alcohol. The result is sweeter, gentler, and entirely appropriate for children and those avoiding alcohol. Glycerin doesn't extract quite as broad a range of constituents as alcohol, but it captures enough to make effective medicine.

Use food-grade vegetable glycerin. For dried herbs, mix glycerin with water - typically three parts glycerin to one part water - to help the extraction. Fresh herbs contain enough water that you can use straight glycerin. Follow the same maceration timeline as tinctures. The resulting glycerite will be sweet and syrupy, with a shelf life of one to two years.

Glycerites are particularly lovely for herbs used with children: chamomile for restlessness, lemon balm for anxiety, elderberry for immune support. The sweetness makes medicine-taking easier for small ones who might otherwise resist.

Oil Preparations: Medicine for the Skin

Infused oils draw out the oil-soluble constituents of herbs - compounds that neither water nor alcohol can reach. These preparations are applied externally, bringing plant medicine directly to skin, muscles, and wounds. From infused oil, we make salves and balms, massage oils and body care. This is the herbal medicine that touches.

❧ Infused Oils: Capturing the Sun

The solar infusion method is the most traditional approach - and there's something deeply satisfying about letting the sun do the work of extraction, the same sun that grew the plant in the first place.

Choose your oil with care. Olive oil is traditional, stable, and good for most purposes. Sweet almond oil is lighter, excellent for massage. Coconut oil brings its own antimicrobial properties. Jojoba - technically a liquid wax rather than an oil - is extremely stable and particularly good for skin care. Each base oil contributes its own qualities to the final medicine.

Here is what matters most: you must use thoroughly dried herbs. Fresh plant material contains water, and water in oil means mold. There is no exception to this rule. If you want to use fresh herbs, wilt them first for a day or two until they're limp and dry, then proceed. But dry is safer, and safer is better when you're learning.

Fill your jar half to three-quarters full with dried herbs. Pour oil over until the herbs are completely submerged. Use a chopstick to release any trapped air bubbles. Make sure everything is covered with at least two inches of oil above.

Place your jar in a sunny window, or outside in direct sunlight if the weather allows. Let it sit for two to four weeks, shaking daily. Watch for any bubbles rising up - this can indicate water content causing fermentation, which means you may need to start over with drier herbs. The oil will slowly take on the color and scent of the plant.

When the infusion is complete, strain through cheesecloth, squeezing well to extract all the oil. Store in dark bottles away from light and heat. A properly made infused oil will last a year or more.

If you don't have weeks to wait - or if the sun isn't cooperating - you can use the heat infusion method instead. Place herbs and oil in a double boiler and heat very gently for two to four hours. The temperature should be low - warm to the touch, never hot enough to fry. Stir occasionally. This achieves in hours what the sun does in weeks, though some herbalists believe the solar method produces superior medicine. Perhaps the sun adds something we can't measure.

The classic herbs for infused oils each bring their own gifts. Calendula is supreme for wound healing and skin soothing. St. John's wort - traditionally infused until the oil turns blood-red - addresses nerve pain, wounds, and bruises. Arnica helps with sore muscles and bruising, though it should never be used on broken skin or taken internally. Comfrey speeds wound healing and soothes sprains. Plantain draws and heals. Lavender relaxes and soothes. As you learn, you'll discover which plants call to you for this kind of work.

❧ Salves and Balms: Oil Made Solid

A salve is simply an infused oil thickened with beeswax - or plant wax, for a vegan preparation - to create a semi-solid that stays where you put it. Salves are practical magic: portable, shelf-stable, ready to apply directly to wounds, sore muscles, dry skin, or wherever healing is needed.

The basic ratio: one ounce of beeswax per cup (eight ounces) of infused oil will give you a standard salve consistency. More wax makes a firmer salve; less wax makes it softer. Climate matters too - you'll want firmer salves in warm climates where they might otherwise melt, softer in cold climates where they might otherwise be hard to apply.

Gently warm your infused oil in a double boiler. Add grated beeswax and stir until completely melted and combined. Test the consistency by dipping a cold spoon into the mixture and letting it cool for a moment - this shows you what the finished salve will feel like. Adjust with more wax or more oil until you're satisfied.

If you want to add essential oils for extra aromatherapy, do so at the very end, when the mixture has cooled slightly but not yet solidified. Vitamin E oil serves as a natural preservative. Shea butter or cocoa butter can be melted in for extra skin nourishment.

Work quickly once everything is melted and combined - salve sets up fast. Pour into small tins or jars. Leave uncovered until completely cooled and solid. Label with herb name, date, and purpose. A well-made salve will last one to two years.

Classic salve combinations to consider: a healing salve with calendula, comfrey, and plantain for wounds and skin repair. A muscle rub with arnica and St. John's wort, perhaps with warming essential oils like ginger or black pepper. A gentle skin soother with calendula, lavender, and chamomile. A drawing salve with plantain and perhaps a touch of activated charcoal or bentonite clay. These are starting points - your own formulas will emerge as you learn what works, what calls to you, what your community needs.

Syrups: Medicine Made Sweet

Syrups are water-based preparations preserved with honey or sugar - ancient medicine that turns bitter herbs palatable and makes dosing children infinitely easier. They're particularly suited for respiratory conditions, where the thick sweetness coats the throat and delivers medicine exactly where it's needed.

Begin by making a strong decoction or infusion - about one-quarter to one-half cup of dried herbs per two cups of water. Simmer or steep until the liquid is reduced to about one cup. Strain very thoroughly; you don't want plant particles in your syrup.

Add honey while the liquid is still warm but not boiling - heat damages honey's beneficial properties. The traditional ratio is equal parts honey to decoction by volume. For longer preservation, use more honey - two parts honey to one part decoction will last considerably longer, though it will also be sweeter. Stir gently until the honey is completely dissolved.

For extended shelf life, you can add a tablespoon or two of brandy or vodka per cup of syrup - this acts as a preservative without significantly changing the character of the medicine. Bottle in clean glass, label, and refrigerate. Without alcohol, your syrup will keep two to three months refrigerated. With alcohol, it can last six months to a year.

Dosing is typically one tablespoon for adults, one teaspoon for children, taken as needed. These are guidelines - adjust based on the herbs used and the situation at hand.

Elderberry syrup is perhaps the most beloved - immune support for cold and flu season, made annually in many herbal households when the elderberries ripen. Thyme honey soothes coughs and fights respiratory infections. Rose hip syrup delivers vitamin C and gentle immune support. Mullein syrup addresses dry, irritating coughs. These syrups become part of the rhythm of household medicine - made seasonally, used when needed, a sweet form of care.

One important note: honey should not be given to children under one year of age due to the risk of infant botulism. For very young children, you can make syrups with sugar instead, though honey's antibacterial properties will be lost.

External Applications: Direct Contact

Sometimes the most effective medicine is the most direct - fresh plant material or herbal preparations applied right where they're needed. These external applications speak immediately to the body, bypassing the digestive system entirely.

Poultices: Plant on Skin

A poultice is the simplest external application - fresh or reconstituted herbs applied directly to the skin. When you chew up a plantain leaf and press it to a bee sting, you're making a poultice. When you mash comfrey leaves onto a sprain, that's a poultice. It's medicine in its most immediate form.

For a fresh poultice, crush, chew, or chop the plant material to release its juices. Apply it directly to the affected area, cover with a clean cloth, and secure with a bandage. Replace every few hours as the poultice dries or warms to body temperature. For a dried herb poultice, mix powdered herbs with enough hot water to make a paste, then apply the same way.

Plantain is the classic poultice herb - drawing, healing, soothing for stings and bites and minor wounds. Comfrey speeds the healing of wounds, sprains, and even fractures, though it should only be used externally. Yarrow helps stop bleeding and heal wounds. Chickweed draws, cools, and relieves itching. These are the herbs you want to know in the field, the plants you can reach for immediately when someone gets hurt.

Compresses: Cloth Soaked in Tea

A compress is a cloth soaked in herbal tea and applied to the skin - a way of delivering water-based medicine externally over a broader area than a poultice allows.

Hot compresses bring blood flow and warmth to an area, helping with sore muscles, congestion, and pain. Make a strong infusion or decoction, soak a clean cloth in the hot liquid, wring out the excess, and apply to the affected area. Replace as it cools. A hot chamomile compress can ease menstrual cramps. A hot ginger compress can warm cold, stiff joints.

Cold compresses reduce inflammation and cool overheated tissues. Make your tea, let it cool completely or refrigerate, then apply the cold cloth. Cold peppermint compresses can help with headaches. Cold witch hazel compresses soothe inflammation and irritation.

Baths and Steams: Immersion

An herbal bath is a whole-body experience - immersion in plant medicine. Make one to two quarts of strong infusion or decoction, strain well, and add to your bath water. Soak for twenty to thirty minutes, letting the medicine absorb through your skin while you breathe in any aromatic compounds. Oat baths soothe itchy, irritated skin. Lavender baths relax body and mind. Ginger baths warm cold bodies and ease muscle aches. Epsom salts can be added for extra mineral absorption and muscle relaxation.

If you don't want to make a tea first, fill a large muslin bag or clean sock with herbs and hang it under the faucet as the tub fills, letting the hot water run through it. Then let the bag float in the bath while you soak, squeezing it occasionally to release more medicine.

Facial or respiratory steams use aromatic herbs to open airways, clear congestion, and bring medicine directly to the sinuses and lungs. Pour boiling water over herbs in a large bowl. Create a tent over your head and the bowl with a towel. Keep your eyes closed - steam can irritate them. Breathe deeply for five to ten minutes. Eucalyptus, thyme, peppermint, and rosemary open the respiratory tract. Chamomile, lavender, and rose are gentler, suited for facial steams and skin care.

Quality and Safety: The Foundation of Good Medicine

Good medicine begins with good materials. The quality of your herbs matters - not in a precious or perfectionist way, but in a practical way. Plants that have been stored too long, dried improperly, or contaminated will not make good medicine, no matter how careful your technique.

When sourcing herbs, look for vibrant color, strong aroma, and no signs of mustiness, mold, or insect damage. Organic herbs, when available, ensure you're not extracting pesticides along with medicine. Dried herbs are best used within a year of harvest for maximum potency - after that, they begin to fade. If you're wildcrafting, harvest from clean areas away from roadsides, agricultural runoff, and industrial contamination. Know your source.

Store dried herbs in airtight containers away from light. Glass jars in a dark cupboard are ideal. Heat, light, and air all degrade plant medicine over time. Label everything with herb name and date acquired, so you know what you have and how long you've had it.

In your medicine-making, cleanliness matters. Use clean equipment. Dry fresh herbs thoroughly before infusing in oil - water causes mold. Never use herbs that have become moldy or smell off. Label everything you make with herb name, date started, method used, and any relevant notes. Check your preparations before use - smell them, look at them. When in doubt, throw it out. Making new medicine is always better than using questionable medicine.

This is not paranoia; it's respect. You're making medicine that will go into bodies - yours, your family's, perhaps eventually your community's. That deserves care.

Dosage: How Much Medicine?

Dosage varies based on who is taking the medicine, which herb is being used, what condition is being addressed, and how concentrated the preparation is. There are no universal formulas here - only guidelines that you adjust through observation and experience.

For teas, a typical dose is three to four cups daily for acute conditions - when you're actively fighting something off. For chronic support or tonic purposes, one to three cups daily is usually sufficient. Some people drink nourishing herb infusions by the quart; others need only a cup to feel the effects.

For tinctures, the standard range is thirty to sixty drops - about one to two milliliters - taken two to four times daily. During acute illness, you might take smaller doses more frequently. Gentle herbs allow for higher doses; potent herbs demand restraint. Always start lower than you think you need and observe. You can always take more; you can't take less.

For children, a common approach: under two years, consult a qualified practitioner rather than experimenting. From two to six years, one-quarter of the adult dose is generally appropriate. From six to twelve, one-half the adult dose. After twelve, most children can take adult doses, adjusted for their size and sensitivity.

Pregnancy and nursing require extra caution - many herbs are contraindicated during these times. If you're pregnant or nursing, stick to the safest herbs only and consult with qualified practitioners before using anything new. This is not the time for experimentation.

Documentation: The Record of Your Learning

Document everything you make. This isn't bureaucracy - it's how you learn, how you improve, how you build a body of knowledge over time.

Record the herb name and part used, the date you started, the method you followed, the measurements and proportions, the type of menstruum (what kind of alcohol, what kind of oil, water temperature). Note the date you finished or strained. Add any observations - how the color changed, what you noticed during the process, how it smelled or tasted, how it turned out.

Then, crucially, document how the medicine *worked*. When you used it, what happened? Was it effective? Would you change anything next time? This closes the learning loop - you're not just making medicine, you're studying it, refining your approach, becoming a better medicine-maker with each preparation.

Over years, these records become invaluable. You can return to successful preparations and replicate them exactly. You can learn from preparations that didn't work as hoped. You build a personal pharmacopoeia grounded in direct experience rather than abstract knowledge.

The Alchemy

You now have the technical knowledge. But remember, making medicine is also alchemy - transformation not just of substances, but of yourself.

Your intention matters. Your presence matters. The care and love you bring to your preparations matters. This is not superstition; it's attention. When you're calm and focused, you measure more accurately, you notice problems earlier, you make better decisions. When you're distracted and hurried, mistakes happen. The medicine reflects the state of the medicine-maker.

As you make medicine, work when you're centered and present. Thank the plants - not as performance, but as genuine acknowledgment of what they're offering. Infuse your preparations with healing intention, not as magic spell but as focused purpose. Notice the transformations happening: the color of alcohol darkening as it draws out plant compounds, the oil slowly shifting hue as the sun does its work, the water becoming tea before your eyes. Stay present with the process rather than rushing to completion.

This is where science meets art meets spirit. This is the alchemy of herbal medicine - the transformation of plant matter into healing, of ingredients into relationship, of practice into wisdom.

Embodied Practice: The Ritual of Making Tea

This practice transforms the simplest preparation - a cup of herbal tea - into a complete meditation, a conversation with a plant, an act of alchemy you can perform daily. It requires only dried herbs, hot water, a cup, and your full attention.

Choose one herb for this practice. Something simple and accessible - chamomile, peppermint, lemon balm, or whatever calls to you from your kitchen or apothecary. You will be with this plant for the next thirty minutes or so. Choose something you want to know better.

Read through the entire practice first. Then set down the book and let the ritual unfold.

❧ Preparing the Space

Clear your workspace. Not obsessively, but enough that you're not surrounded by distraction. Turn off your phone or put it in another room. You are creating a container for attention.

Set out what you'll need: your kettle or pot of water, your cup or teapot, your dried herb, something to cover the tea while it steeps. A timer if you want one, though your body can learn to track time too.

Before you begin, take three slow breaths. Feel your feet on the floor. Arrive fully in your body, in this moment, in this kitchen that is about to become a laboratory of transformation.

❧ Meeting the Plant

Pick up the jar or bag that holds your herb. Before you open it, hold it in your hands for a moment. Consider what you're holding: a plant that grew from seed, that was tended or wild-harvested, that was dried and stored and transported to reach you. Consider the journey this medicine has already taken.

Open the container and bring it to your nose. Inhale slowly. What do you notice? Not just "it smells like chamomile" - but what is the *quality* of this scent? Is it bright or muted? Sweet or bitter? Does it rise quickly or unfold slowly? What happens in your body as you breathe it in?

Look at the dried herb. Notice its color, texture, form. If it's flowers, can you see the original shape of the blossom? If it's leaves, how did the drying change them? Touch the herbs gently. Feel their texture against your fingertips.

This is the being you're about to enter into conversation with. Take a moment to acknowledge that.

❧ The Alchemy of Water

As you heat your water, stay present. Watch the kettle or pot. Listen to the sounds it makes as the water warms - the quiet settling, the first whisper of movement, the building rumble, finally the full boil.

Consider what is happening: you are adding energy to water, making its molecules move faster, preparing it to become a solvent, a medium of extraction. Heat is transformation. This is alchemy in its most literal form.

While the water heats, measure your herb. One tablespoon per cup - a rough measure, adjusted by your growing intuition. Place the herbs in your cup or teapot. Arrange them or leave them loose. There's no wrong way.

❧ The Moment of Meeting

When the water has boiled, let it rest for just a moment - a breath, no more. Then pour it over the herbs.

Watch this moment carefully. This is the meeting - water and plant, heat and matter, solvent and solute coming together.

See how the herbs respond to the water. Do they float or sink? Do they release color immediately, or hold back? Does steam carry fragrance to your nose? Watch the water begin to change color as it draws the plant's essence into itself.

Cover your tea. This is important - the cover keeps the volatile oils from escaping, holds the medicine in. Watch the condensation form on the lid or plate. That's plant medicine rising with the steam and being returned to your cup.

❧ The Waiting

Now you wait. Ten to fifteen minutes for medicinal strength - longer than a casual cup of tea, long enough that you might be tempted to wander off and do something else.

Stay. This is the practice.

Use this time to be still. You can close your eyes and simply breathe. You can watch the tea steep, noticing how the color deepens over time. You can place your hands around the cup or pot, feeling the warmth, feeling the transformation happening inside.

Consider: while you wait, the water is doing invisible work. It's entering the cells of the dried plant, dissolving compounds, carrying them into solution. The plant is giving its medicine to the water. The water is becoming something new - no longer just water, not yet tea, transforming in the between.

This is alchemy. This is what you're learning to do with attention: to be present for transformation.

❧ Receiving the Medicine

When the time has passed, remove the cover. A rush of fragrant steam may rise - breathe it in. This too is medicine.

If you need to strain, do so slowly, watching the liquid pour, noticing its color. If the herbs remain in the cup, that's fine too - they'll settle to the bottom.

Before you drink, hold the cup in your hands. Feel its warmth. Bring it to your nose and inhale again - the scent will be different now, transformed by the steeping. Look at the color. This is your medicine.

If you wish, speak a word of thanks - to the plant, to the water, to the process that brought this cup into being. Not performance, just acknowledgment.

Then drink.

Drink slowly. Let the tea move over your tongue, noticing the taste - not just naming it, but feeling it. Notice the temperature as it moves down your throat. Feel it settling into your belly.

As you continue to drink, notice what begins to happen in your body. Does the warmth spread? Does your breathing change? Does something in you relax, or wake up? This is the plant working. This is what you made.

❧ Closing

When the cup is empty - or when you've drunk as much as feels right - take a moment before you rush back to life.

Notice how you feel now, compared to before you began. What shifted? What do you know now about this plant that you didn't know before?

If you keep a journal, this is a good time to write a few notes - not an essay, just impressions. The color of the tea. The taste. How it made you feel. Anything that surprised you. These notes become part of your growing materia medica, your record of relationship.

The spent herbs can go to compost, returning to the earth that grew them. The cup can be washed and put away. The practice is complete.

But here is the invitation: do this again tomorrow. And the next day. With the same herb, or with different ones. Let making tea become a daily practice, a ritual of attention, a way of showing up for the plants and for yourself.

Every cup of tea is an opportunity for alchemy. Every cup is a conversation. Every cup is medicine - if you're present for it.

Reflection Questions

1. Which preparation method calls to you most strongly? What draws you to it - practicality, aesthetics, intuition, something else?

2. What makes you nervous about making medicine? How might you address those concerns while still moving forward?

3. What herbs are you most eager to work with first? What draws you to them?

. . .

4. How does it feel to think of yourself as someone who makes medicine? What identity shifts might this require?

5. What did you notice during the tea-making practice? What surprised you about bringing full attention to something so ordinary?

Welcome to the medicine-making path.
Your hands hold healing.
Go create.

Chapter 4
Reading the Body
Plant Allies for Different Tissues & States

Learning to See

YOU'VE LEARNED the language of plants through preparation. You've begun to sense their energetics through your own body. Now comes the other half of the conversation: learning to read the language of the body itself.

This is where herbalism becomes truly effective. It's not about memorizing which herb treats which symptom - that approach, while tempting in its simplicity, misses the deeper truth. Bodies are not machines with interchangeable parts. Each person is a unique landscape, and the same symptom can arise from entirely different terrain.

What you're learning instead is pattern recognition - the ability to see whether tissue is hot or cold, dry or damp, tense or lax. To understand not just *what* is happening, but *why*. And from that understanding, to match the right plant ally to the actual condition, not just the surface complaint.

This chapter introduces the six primary tissue states - the fundamental patterns that show up again and again across different bodies and different systems. But remember: the real learning comes from observing yourself and others, noticing patterns, developing your eye and your intuition. The map is here. The territory is everywhere around you, waiting to be read.

Beyond Symptom Matching

Many beginning herbalists want a simple list: this herb for that symptom. Elderberry for colds. Valerian for sleep. Chamomile for digestion. And there's a place for that kind of knowledge - it gets you started; it gives you something to work with.

But bodies are complex. The same symptom can arise from entirely different root causes, and each requires different medicine.

Consider someone who comes to you saying, "I'm tired." Such a simple complaint - and yet it could mean so many things. Perhaps their reserves are depleted, and they need nourishing tonics to rebuild what has been spent. Perhaps their circulation is sluggish, and they need warming stimulants to get energy moving. Perhaps they're holding so much tension that their body is exhausting itself just staying contracted, and they need calming nervines to let go. Perhaps inflammation is consuming their energy, requiring cooling anti-inflammatories. Perhaps their digestion is compromised and they're simply not absorbing nutrients from their food.

Each of these patterns requires different herbs. Giving warming stimulants to someone with inflammation will make things worse. Giving cooling herbs to someone who's already cold and depleted will deepen their exhaustion. The symptom is the same - tiredness - but the medicine must match the pattern underneath.

This is why we learn to see tissue states: to look beneath the surface symptom to the actual condition of the tissues and systems. This is what allows herbalism to be precise rather than merely hopeful.

THE SIX PRIMARY TISSUE STATES

These six patterns appear throughout the body in different systems - digestive, respiratory, nervous, reproductive, skin. Learning to recognize them is fundamental to effective herbalism. They are not diseases to diagnose but landscapes to recognize, each calling for its own kind of care.

❧ Heat and Inflammation: The Body on Fire

You recognize heat by its signs: redness that shows where blood has rushed in, warmth you can feel when you touch the skin, swelling where fluid has gathered, pain that often has a burning or throbbing quality. The person may be restless, irritable, thirsty for cold drinks. Their pulse tends to be rapid. Their tongue, if you look, is often red, sometimes with a yellow coating that indicates heat has been present for a while.

Heat arises from many sources. Acute infection or injury will create it - this is the body's inflammatory response doing its protective work. Chronic inflammation can simmer in joints, digestive tract, or skin for years. Excess metabolic activity generates heat. Chronic stress creates heat in the body, as anyone who has ever felt anger flush their face knows. A diet high in inflammatory foods - sugar, processed oils, excessive alcohol - stokes internal fire.

What does heat need? Cooling. Anti-inflammatory herbs that calm the fire without suppressing the body's wisdom. Demulcent herbs that soothe and coat irritated tissues. Support for lymphatic drainage, which helps clear the debris of inflammation. Rest, hydration, cooling foods. And often, a reduction in whatever inputs are feeding the flames.

The plant allies for heat include peppermint, which cools and disperses; chamomile, which calms inflammation gently; calendula, which cools while supporting lymphatic movement and healing; violet leaf, which is both cooling and moistening; chickweed, which draws heat out; and plantain, which cools while healing and fighting infection. These are the herbs you reach for when something is red, hot, swollen, angry.

Picture this pattern: red, hot, swollen eczema patches that itch and burn. Hot to the touch, worse with stress and in warm weather. This is heat calling for cooling, soothing medicine.

❧ Cold and Stagnation: The Body Slowed

Cold is heat's opposite - and you recognize it by opposite signs. Paleness where there should be healthy color. Coldness to the touch, especially in the hands and feet. Sluggish circulation that leaves the extremities bloodless. Low energy that makes everything feel effortful. Slow metabolism that holds onto weight. A craving for warmth - warm foods, warm drinks, warm environments. The tongue, if you look, is pale and often swollen, with tooth marks along the edges where it presses against the teeth.

Cold comes from poor circulation, from low metabolic activity, from lack of movement. It comes from living in cold climates without enough warmth, from thyroid imbalances that slow everything down, from chronic fatigue that has banked the body's fires. Sometimes it's constitutional - some people simply run cold, and have all their lives.

What does cold need? Warmth. Stimulating herbs that stoke the internal fire. Circulatory support that gets blood moving to the periphery. Movement itself - physical and energetic. Warming foods, adequate protein for fuel. Heat therapy, exercise, anything that generates warmth from within.

The plant allies for cold include ginger, our great warming disperser; cinnamon, which warms sweetly and supports circulation; cayenne, which is hot and stimulating and moves blood powerfully; rosemary, which warms while bringing mental clarity; black pepper, which sparks digestive fire; and garlic, which warms while fighting infection. These are the herbs that bring heat back to a body that has grown too cold.

Picture this pattern: always cold, especially in the hands and feet. Low energy, pale complexion, slow digestion. Feels better with warmth, worse in winter. This is cold calling for warming, stimulating medicine.

❧ Dryness and Atrophy: The Body Parched

Dryness shows itself everywhere the body needs moisture. Dry skin that cracks and flakes. Dry lips that chap easily. Dry mucous membranes - in the mouth, the eyes, the respiratory tract, the digestive system. Constipation with hard, dry stools that are difficult to pass. A dry cough with little or no mucus. Constant thirst that drinking doesn't quite satisfy. Brittle hair that breaks, brittle nails that split. Sometimes muscle wasting and thinness, as if the body is drying out from the inside. The tongue, if you look, is dry and thin, often with cracks running across its surface.

Dryness arises from dehydration, certainly, but also from lack of healthy fats in the diet. It can come from excessive use of drying herbs or drying foods - too much caffeine, too much astringent tea. Aging naturally brings dryness as tissues lose their ability to hold moisture. Chronic stress depletes the fluids of the body - we speak of "burning out" for a reason. Hot, dry climates contribute. So does any condition that uses up the body's reserves faster than they can be replenished.

What does dryness need? Moisture. Demulcent herbs that coat and soothe. Nourishing herbs that rebuild what has been depleted. Healthy fats in the diet - omega-3s, olive oil, avocado. Adequate hydration, though water alone often isn't enough when dryness is deep. Rest and restoration, time for the body to rebuild its reserves.

The plant allies for dryness include marshmallow root, deeply moistening and demulcent; slippery elm, which soothes and coats; licorice root, which moistens while building strength; violet leaf, cooling and moistening together; milky oat tops, profoundly nourishing and restorative; and flax seed, moistening and rich in omega-3s. These are the herbs that bring water back to parched ground.

Picture this pattern: dry skin, dry cough, constipation, thinning hair. Drinks water constantly but still feels parched. This is dryness calling for moistening, nourishing medicine.

❧ Dampness and Excess: The Body Waterlogged

Dampness is dryness's opposite - too much fluid where there should be free flow. You see it as edema, water retention that leaves ankles puffy and faces swollen. Excessive mucus production - in the sinuses, the lungs, the digestive tract. Loose stools, bloating, a sense of heaviness in the belly. A sluggish, heavy feeling throughout the body, as if moving through water. Weight gain, especially water weight that fluctuates. The tongue, if you look, has a thick white coating, and is often swollen and puffy with tooth marks at the edges.

Dampness accumulates when the body's drainage systems aren't working well. Poor lymphatic flow allows fluid to pool. Sluggish digestion fails to transform what we eat and drink. A diet heavy in damp-forming foods - dairy, sugar, refined flour, excessive raw and cold foods - contributes more moisture than the body can process. Lack of movement lets everything stagnate. What traditional Chinese medicine calls weak spleen energy - the digestive fire that transforms food into energy - allows dampness to accumulate rather than be metabolized.

What does dampness need? Drying. Astringent herbs that tighten and tone waterlogged tissues. Lymphatic movers that get stagnant fluid flowing again. Digestive bitters that wake up sluggish digestion. Movement and sweating to release excess through the skin. A reduction in damp-forming foods, at least until balance is restored.

The plant allies for dampness include cleavers, which drains lymphatic congestion; red clover, alterative and lymphatic; burdock root, which moves stagnation through the liver and lymph; dandelion root, bitter and gently diuretic; nettles, drying and nutritive simultaneously; and yarrow, astringent and able to open the pores for sweating. These are the herbs that help the body release what it's been holding.

Picture this pattern: bloating, water retention, excessive mucus, feeling heavy and sluggish. Puffy face and ankles. This is dampness calling for drying, moving medicine.

❧ Tension and Spasm: The Body Gripped

Tension is the body held tight - muscles contracted that should be relaxed, tissues gripped that should be soft. You see it in chronic muscle tension, in cramping, in headaches that come from clenched jaws and hunched shoulders. In digestive cramping and the spasms of irritable bowel. In anxiety that lives in the body as tightness, in restlessness that can't settle, in the inability to relax even when rest is desperately needed. When you touch tissue that's in a tension state, it feels tight, contracted, sometimes almost rigid.

Tension arises most often from chronic stress - the body's fight-or-flight response that never fully releases. Mineral deficiencies contribute, especially magnesium and calcium, which muscles need to relax. Overwork and insufficient rest keep the body in a contracted state. Trauma, whether physical or emotional, can lock tension into tissues for years. Excessive stimulant use - too much caffeine, for instance - keeps the nervous system wound tight.

What does tension need? Relaxation. Antispasmodic herbs that release cramped muscles. Nervines that calm the nervous system driving the contraction. Minerals, especially magnesium. Rest and downtime, nervous system support. Breath work, which can directly release held tension. Gentle movement like yoga that teaches the body to let go. Warm baths that coax muscles to soften.

The plant allies for tension include valerian, strongly antispasmodic and sedating; cramp bark, which relaxes smooth muscle throughout the body; passionflower, nervine and antispasmodic together; skullcap, which deeply relaxes the nervous system; chamomile, gently antispasmodic and calming; and lemon balm, which eases both nervous tension and digestive spasm. These are the herbs that teach the body it's safe to let go.

Picture this pattern: chronic muscle tension, frequent headaches, digestive cramping, difficulty sleeping because the body can't unwind. This is tension calling for relaxing, antispasmodic medicine.

Laxity and Weakness: The Body Loosened

Laxity is tension's opposite - tissue that has lost its tone, structure that no longer holds. You see it as sagging tissue, as prolapse where organs descend from their proper position - uterus, bladder, rectum. As varicose veins and hemorrhoids where blood vessels have lost their integrity. As loose, hypermobile joints that bend too far. As easy bruising where capillaries break under the slightest pressure. Weak muscle tone, a body that feels unsupported from within. The tongue, if you look, is often pale and flabby.

Laxity comes from tissue damage or trauma that has stretched things beyond their capacity to return. From aging and the natural loss of collagen that comes with time. From chronic nutritional deficiency - the body can't maintain structure without the materials to build it. From lack of physical conditioning, muscles that have never developed strength. From multiple pregnancies and births that have stressed pelvic tissues. Sometimes from genetic factors, as in conditions like Ehlers-Danlos syndrome.

What does laxity need? Toning. Astringent herbs that tighten and firm tissue. Tonifying herbs that strengthen over time. Collagen-building nutrients - vitamin C, silica, copper, the raw materials of structural tissue. Strength training, gentle resistance exercise that rebuilds muscle tone. Adequate protein for repair.

The plant allies for laxity include witch hazel, astringent for veins and tissue; oak bark, strongly astringent; raspberry leaf, a classic uterine tonic with astringent properties; horsetail, rich in silica for connective tissue support; nettles, mineral-rich and tonifying; and lady's mantle, astringent and particularly supportive for women. These are the herbs that help rebuild structure where it has weakened.

Picture this pattern: varicose veins, hemorrhoids, weak pelvic floor, easy bruising. Tissues that feel loose and unsupported. This is laxity calling for astringent, tonifying medicine.

ASSESSMENT SKILLS: LEARNING TO SEE PATTERNS

Effective herbalism requires observation and inquiry - learning to see what is actually happening rather than just hearing a symptom and reaching for a protocol. You're not diagnosing disease; that is the work of licensed medical professionals. What you're doing is assessing tissue states and patterns to guide your herb selection. This is a different skill, and one that takes time to develop.

There are four basic tools you'll use: observation, inquiry, palpation, and pattern recognition. Each offers different information. Together, they build a picture.

❧ Observation: What Can You See?

Before you ask a single question, you can learn a great deal simply by looking. Notice the general appearance - skin color and tone, energy level and vitality, posture and how someone moves through space, body type and build, overall presence. A person's body tells a story before they ever open their mouth.

The tongue is particularly revealing - a window into the body's internal state that traditional systems have used for thousands of years. Its color tells you about heat and cold: a pale tongue suggests cold or deficiency, a normal pink indicates balance, a red tongue shows heat, a purple or bluish tongue indicates stagnation and poor circulation. Its coating tells you about digestion and dampness: no coating suggests dryness, a thin white coat is normal or slightly cold, a thick white coat indicates dampness, a yellow coat indicates heat. Its shape tells you about fluid balance: a thin tongue suggests deficiency and dryness, a swollen tongue with tooth marks indicates dampness, cracks often indicate heat or long-standing dryness. Its moisture tells you about hydration: a dry tongue speaks of dehydration or heat, excessive wetness indicates dampness.

Look also at the nails - ridges can indicate periods of stress or nutritional deficiency, brittleness suggests dryness, healthy smooth nails reflect good nutrition and balance. Look at the hair - thin and dry often indicates deficiency, oily indicates excess, premature graying can suggest deep depletion. Look at the eyes - bright and clear reflects vitality, dull suggests depletion, bloodshot shows heat or inflammation. Look at the skin quality throughout - its texture, color, moisture. Everything is information.

❧ Inquiry: What Does the Person Report?

Observation gives you one layer. Inquiry gives you another - the person's own experience of their body, which only they can report.

Ask open-ended questions about energy: How does your energy move through the day? When do you feel most vital, most depleted? How is your sleep - do you fall asleep easily, stay asleep, wake rested? These questions reveal patterns of deficiency or excess, tension or depletion.

Ask about temperature: Do you tend to run hot or cold? Do you prefer warm drinks or cold ones? How do different temperatures affect how you feel? These questions directly reveal the hot/cold pattern.

Ask about digestion: How is your digestion overall? What is your appetite like? Tell me about your bowel movements - frequency, consistency, ease. Digestion is central to health, and these questions reveal dampness, dryness, heat, cold, tension - almost every pattern shows up in the gut.

Ask about emotional and mental states: How do you respond to stress? What has your mood been like lately? Do you tend toward anxiety, depression, calm, agitation? The mind and body are not separate; emotional patterns often mirror and influence physical ones.

Ask about patterns: Are your symptoms worse with heat or cold? Better with rest or movement? Affected by weather, seasons, stress? How long has this been going on - is it recent or long-standing? These questions help you see how the condition behaves, which points to its nature.

Listen not just for facts but for patterns. The same condition will manifest differently in different constitutional types. Your job is to hear beneath the words to the terrain underneath.

❧ Palpation: What Can You Feel?

With appropriate permission and respect for boundaries, touch provides another layer of information that no other sense can gather.

Feel for temperature - is the skin warm or cool? Are some areas warmer than others? Compare hands to feet, forehead to belly. Temperature variations tell you where heat is accumulating or where circulation is failing to reach.

Feel for moisture - is the skin dry, normal, or clammy with sweat? What is the sweating pattern? Dampness and dryness both show up in the skin.

Feel for tissue quality - is there tension or relaxation? Does tissue feel tight and congested, boggy and waterlogged, or depleted and thin? Are there specific areas of heat or cold? The quality of tissue under your hands tells you about its state.

The areas most commonly assessed include the abdomen, where you can feel tension, tenderness, temperature, and sometimes hear bowel sounds; the neck and shoulders, where tension and heat often accumulate; and the extremities, where temperature and circulation quality are most obvious. If you're trained in pulse assessment, the pulse offers rich information about energy, heat, cold, and strength - but this requires specific study to develop.

❧ Pattern Recognition: What's the Underlying State?

Now you combine all your observations into an overall pattern. This is where the skill becomes art - taking disparate pieces of information and seeing the coherent picture underneath.

Ask yourself the primary questions: Is this primarily hot or cold? Dry or damp? Tense or lax? Is it excess - too much of something - or deficiency - not enough? Is it acute, happening right now, or chronic, present for a long time?

Let's see this in action. A person presents with pale complexion, cold hands and feet, sluggish digestion, low energy, and tells you they feel better with warmth and crave hot drinks. This adds up to a clear pattern: cold and stagnation. They need warming, stimulating herbs.

Another person presents with red, inflamed skin, reports thirst and irritability, has a rapid pulse and seems restless. Their tongue is red with a yellow coating. This is a heat and inflammation pattern. They need cooling, anti-inflammatory herbs.

A third person has dry skin, a dry cough, constipation, constant thirst, and brittle hair. Their tongue is dry and cracked. This is a dryness pattern. They need moistening, demulcent herbs.

Once you identify the tissue state, you match it with herbs of appropriate energetics. The fundamental principle: opposite energetics tend to balance each other. Hot conditions need cooling herbs. Cold conditions need warming herbs. Dry conditions need moistening herbs. Damp conditions need drying herbs. Tense conditions need relaxing herbs. Lax conditions need tonifying herbs.

This isn't rigid - sometimes you work with a condition rather than against it - but it's a reliable starting point. Trust the pattern. Match the plant to the person, not just to the symptom.

Learning Through Cases

Let's work through some examples to see this pattern recognition in practice. These are composites, simplified for teaching, but they illustrate how to think.

Sarah: Digestive Troubles

Sarah comes with digestive complaints - bloating after meals, alternating constipation and loose stools, abdominal cramping that's clearly worse when she's stressed. She describes anxiety, especially around food, as if eating itself has become a source of worry. Her tongue is pale with slight tooth marks. When you ask what makes it better, she says warmth on her belly helps.

What patterns do you see? The cramping and the stress connection point to tension as a primary pattern - her nervous system is driving digestive spasm. The bloating and loose stools suggest some dampness. The pale tongue and relief from warmth suggest some cold. This is a picture of a sensitive digestive system being gripped by nervous tension, with some dampness and cold underneath.

What does she need? Calming antispasmodics that will release the grip. Gentle digestive support that won't overwhelm a sensitive system. Some warming to address the cold signs. Herbs like chamomile, which is both calming and gently digestive; lemon balm, which eases both anxiety and digestive spasm; fennel, which reduces gas and brings gentle warmth; small amounts of ginger for warmth and digestive support; perhaps gentle bitters like dandelion before meals to wake up digestive capacity.

This approach addresses the nervous system component driving the tension, supports digestive function without being harsh, is gentle enough for a sensitive system, and includes the warming element to address cold signs. We're treating Sarah's pattern, not just her symptoms.

Michael: Chronic Fatigue

Michael's main complaint is exhaustion. He's always cold, especially in his hands and feet. His energy is lowest in the morning - he can barely get going. His circulation seems poor. He craves warm foods and drinks, has no appetite in the morning, and his tongue is pale with a weak pulse. Interestingly, he says he feels better once he gets moving - movement seems to help, if he can just get started.

What patterns emerge? This is a clear picture of cold and stagnation - the coldness, the poor circulation, the craving for warmth, the pale tongue, the weakness. There's also deficiency underneath - his reserves are depleted, not just stuck. The fact that movement helps suggests the cold is creating stagnation that can be shifted, not complete depletion.

What does Michael need? Warming circulatory support to get energy moving to the periphery. Nourishing tonics to rebuild the reserves underneath. Herbs like ginger for warming and circulation; cinnamon, which warms sweetly and supports energy; astragalus, an immune and energy tonic that's gently warming; nettles for deep mineral nourishment; hawthorn for cardiovascular support. Warming bone broths with herbs would be excellent medicine for Michael - nourishment and warmth together.

This approach increases circulation and warmth, builds the underlying deficiency, supports long-term vitality rather than just giving a quick stimulant lift, and addresses root causes rather than just symptoms.

Jennifer: Skin Inflammation

Jennifer has eczema - red, hot, itchy patches that drive her to distraction. The eczema is clearly worse with stress and in hot weather. She's thirsty, craves cold drinks, and sleeps restlessly. Her tongue is red with a yellow coating. Some patches are rough and dry amidst all the inflammation - heat and dryness together.

What patterns do you see? This is primarily heat and inflammation - the redness, the heat, the itching, the thirst, the red tongue with yellow coating. But there's also dryness in those rough patches - inflammation has dried out some tissue. And stress is clearly a trigger, so the nervous system is involved.

What does Jennifer need? Cooling anti-inflammatories to calm the heat. Moistening demulcents for the dry patches. Lymphatic support to help drain inflammatory debris. Nervous system support for the stress component. Internally: calendula for cooling, anti-inflammatory, and lymphatic support; violet leaf for cooling and moistening; marshmallow root for deep moistening; burdock root as an alterative that cools and clears; chamomile for stress and sleep. Topically: calendula-infused oil or salve, chickweed poultice for acute flares.

Dietary changes would also help Jennifer - reducing inflammatory foods like sugar, dairy, and processed foods; increasing cooling foods like cucumber, watermelon, and leafy greens; ensuring adequate hydration and healthy fats. We're cooling the inflammation systemically and topically, moistening the dry tissue, supporting lymphatic drainage, and addressing the stress component. The whole pattern.

Developing Your Clinical Eye

This is how you develop the ability to think like a clinical herbalist: through practice, observation, and humility.

Observe constantly. Notice people's coloring, their energy, how they carry themselves. Practice tongue observation - look at your own tongue daily, and you'll begin to see how it changes with your state. Notice patterns in yourself and others, not to diagnose but to develop your eye.

Ask good questions. Practice taking case histories with friends who are willing to be your guinea pigs. Learn to listen deeply - not just to the words, but to what lives beneath them. Notice what people say and what they don't say.

Think in patterns, not symptoms. Train yourself to ask: Is this hot or cold? Dry or damp? Tense or lax? Excess or deficiency? Let these questions become automatic, a lens through which you see every presentation.

Match energetics to patterns. Cooling herbs for heat. Warming herbs for cold. And so on. Let the pattern tell you what kind of medicine is needed, then choose specific herbs that fit.

Document and learn. Keep notes on what you observe, what you try, what works and what doesn't. Every person you work with teaches you something. Let your experience accumulate into wisdom.

And stay humble. You are always learning. Bodies are complex. Sometimes patterns aren't clear. It's okay to say "I don't know." It's okay to refer out when something is beyond your skill. Humility is not weakness - it's the ground from which wisdom grows.

Knowing Your Limits

As an herbalist, knowing your scope and limits is as important as knowing your herbs. You can offer tremendous support - and you can also get out of your depth. Wisdom lies in knowing the difference.

Refer to medical professionals when symptoms are severe or worsening, when there's any possibility of serious pathology, in emergency situations like chest pain or severe bleeding, when diagnosis is needed (you assess patterns, not diseases), when pharmaceutical intervention may be necessary, for pregnancy complications, for mental health crises, or for anything that feels beyond your training. You can work alongside medical care, but know when it's needed.

There is no shame in referring. There is only wisdom in knowing what you can hold and what requires other hands. The best herbalists are those who know their limits as well as their gifts.

Embodied Practice: Mapping Your Inner Terrain

This practice teaches you to read your body's signals from the inside out - to sense tissue states through direct felt experience rather than external observation. It requires nothing but a quiet place, a comfortable position, and your full attention. Over time, this practice trains your body awareness so deeply that you begin to sense patterns in yourself instantly, and eventually to perceive them in others through presence and intuition.

The body is always communicating. We simply haven't been taught to listen. This practice is a way of learning the language your body has been speaking all along - a language of warmth and coolness, moisture and dryness, tension and ease. When you can feel these qualities in yourself, you understand them in a way no textbook can teach.

Read through the entire practice first. Then find a quiet space, lie down or sit comfortably, and let the journey unfold.

❧ Arriving

Find a comfortable position - lying down is ideal, but sitting works if that's more accessible. Close your eyes. Let your body be held by whatever surface supports you. There is nothing to do right now except arrive.

Take several slow breaths, letting each exhale be longer than the inhale. With each breath out, feel yourself settling more deeply into stillness. Let your jaw soften. Let your shoulders release. Let your belly be soft.

You are about to take a journey through your own landscape. There is nothing to fix, nothing to change. You are simply here to notice, to witness, to learn the terrain.

❧ Sensing Temperature

Begin by sensing temperature throughout your body. Not thinking about whether you're hot or cold - actually feeling it, from the inside.

Start with your feet. What is the temperature there? Not what your mind thinks it should be, but what you actually sense. Are your feet warm, cool, cold? Is there any difference between one foot and the other? Just notice.

Move your attention slowly up through your legs. What temperature do you feel in your calves, your knees, your thighs? Is the warmth even, or does it vary? Are there areas that feel particularly cool, or particularly warm?

Bring your attention to your pelvis and belly. This is often where core warmth lives - or where you notice its absence. Does your belly feel warm, vital? Or cool, perhaps sluggish? What about your lower back?

Move up through your chest and heart area. What temperature do you sense there? Is there warmth radiating outward, or does it feel contained, cool?

Notice your hands. Hands and feet often tell the truth about circulation - warm hands suggest warmth and good flow; cold hands can indicate that heat isn't reaching the periphery.

Finally, notice your head and face. Is there warmth there? Some people carry heat in their heads - flushed, warm, perhaps with a tendency toward headaches. Others feel cool throughout.

What did you discover? Do you tend toward warmth or coolness overall? Are there areas where heat accumulates, or areas that feel consistently cold? This is your temperature pattern - the first layer of your inner terrain.

❧ Sensing Moisture

Now shift your attention to moisture - the quality of fluidity or dryness in your tissues.

Begin with your mouth. Without moving, just sense - does your mouth feel moist and comfortable? Dry, perhaps sticky? Notice your lips, your throat. Is there a sense of adequate moisture, or of thirst?

Move your attention to your skin - you can sense it from the inside. Does your skin feel supple, nourished? Or dry, perhaps tight? Notice areas where skin tends toward dryness - hands, face, shins - and areas that stay more moist.

Sense into your joints. Joints need fluid to move smoothly. Do yours feel lubricated, easy? Or dry, stiff, perhaps crackly? Notice your shoulders, your hips, your knees.

Notice your belly and digestive area. Is there a sense of moisture there - perhaps too much, a boggy or heavy feeling? Or does it feel dry, perhaps with a sense of constraint or stuckness?

You might also notice areas that feel congested - where fluid seems to be pooling or not moving well. Puffiness, heaviness, a sense of stagnation. This is dampness accumulating.

What did you discover? Do you tend toward dryness - parched tissues that want nourishment? Or toward dampness - fluids accumulating, heaviness, congestion? Or perhaps different patterns in different areas?

❧ Sensing Tension and Ease

Now bring your attention to the quality of tension or relaxation in your tissues.

Begin with your face. Is your jaw clenched or soft? Your forehead - smooth or furrowed, even subtly? What about the tiny muscles around your eyes?

Notice your neck and shoulders - common places where tension accumulates. Are they gripped, held, braced? Or soft, released, at ease? Don't try to change anything. Just notice what is.

Move your attention down through your back. The muscles along your spine, your lower back, your mid-back between the shoulder blades. Is there gripping? Holding? Or a sense of softness and support?

Notice your belly. The belly is a profound indicator of our state - when we feel safe, the belly is soft. When we're anxious or braced against life, the belly tightens. What do you feel there?

Sense your pelvic floor - the muscles at the base of your torso. This is another area that holds tension we may not be aware of. Is there gripping there, or ease?

Finally, notice your hands. Are they curled, clenched, ready for action? Or open, soft, receptive?

What did you discover? Do you hold chronic tension - the body gripped against something, even when there's no immediate threat? Or do you tend toward laxity - tissue that's lost its tone, feels unsupported, maybe too loose? Most of us carry some of each in different places.

❧ Sensing Vitality

Now sense something more subtle - the quality of vitality, of life force, moving through you.

This isn't about thinking about your energy level - it's about feeling the actual sense of aliveness in your tissues. Some people feel this as a subtle hum or vibration. Others sense it as warmth, or flow, or simply presence.

Notice where vitality feels strongest in your body. Your heart? Your belly? Your hands? Where does life seem to concentrate?

Notice where vitality feels diminished - areas that seem quiet, dim, less alive. These might be places of depletion, stagnation, or simply less awareness.

Notice the overall quality. Does your vitality feel robust today, or depleted? Flowing freely, or stuck? Steady, or fluctuating?

This is perhaps the most important thing to sense - the quality of life force in your own body. It tells you whether you're resourced or depleted, whether you need stimulation or rest, building up or letting go.

❧ Integrating

Now let go of any focused attention and simply rest in awareness of your whole body at once. Let all the information you've gathered settle into a felt sense of your current state.

If you were to describe your inner terrain today in terms of the tissue states, what would you say? Are you running hot or cold? Dry or damp? Tense or lax? Vital or depleted? Perhaps a combination - tense and cold, or hot and dry, or damp and depleted?

There is no right answer. There is only what is true for you, today, in this moment. Tomorrow might be different. This is simply a snapshot of your terrain right now.

If an herb comes to mind - something your body seems to be asking for - notice that. Your body knows what it needs. Sometimes, in the quiet of deep listening, it will tell you.

❧ Returning

When you feel complete, begin to bring small movements back to your body. Wiggle your fingers and toes. Take a deeper breath. Perhaps stretch gently.

Open your eyes slowly. Take a moment before you rise. Let the information you gathered settle into your body's knowing.

If you keep a journal, now is a good time to write a few notes - not an analysis, just what you noticed. Today I felt: cool in my extremities, dry in my mouth and skin, tension in my shoulders, low vitality overall. Or whatever is true for you.

❧ Making This a Practice

This body scan can become a regular practice - daily, weekly, or whenever you want to check in with your inner terrain. Over time, you'll notice patterns. Perhaps you always run cold. Perhaps stress shows up as tension in your belly before you're consciously aware of being stressed. Perhaps dryness accumulates in winter and dampness in spring.

As you become fluent in sensing your own body, you'll find this awareness extends outward. You'll begin to sense the quality of others' energy when you're with them - not through analysis, but through a kind of resonance. This is how intuitive assessment develops: not by learning rules, but by building such deep familiarity with your own terrain that you can recognize the same landscapes in others.

Your body is your first patient, your lifelong teacher, your most honest mirror. Learn to read it, and you learn to read the language all bodies speak.

Reflection Questions

1. What is your primary tissue state tendency right now? What signs lead you to this assessment?

2. How does it feel to shift from "herb for symptom" thinking to pattern recognition? What opens up? What feels challenging?

3. Which tissue state is easiest for you to recognize? Which is hardest? Why might that be?

4. What did you notice when you began observing your own tongue? What patterns emerged over time?

5. What questions remain for you about reading the body's signals? What do you want to explore further?

The body speaks. The plants answer.
You are learning to be the bridge between them.
Practice observing. Practice listening. The patterns will reveal themselves.

Part Two
The Wheel of the Year

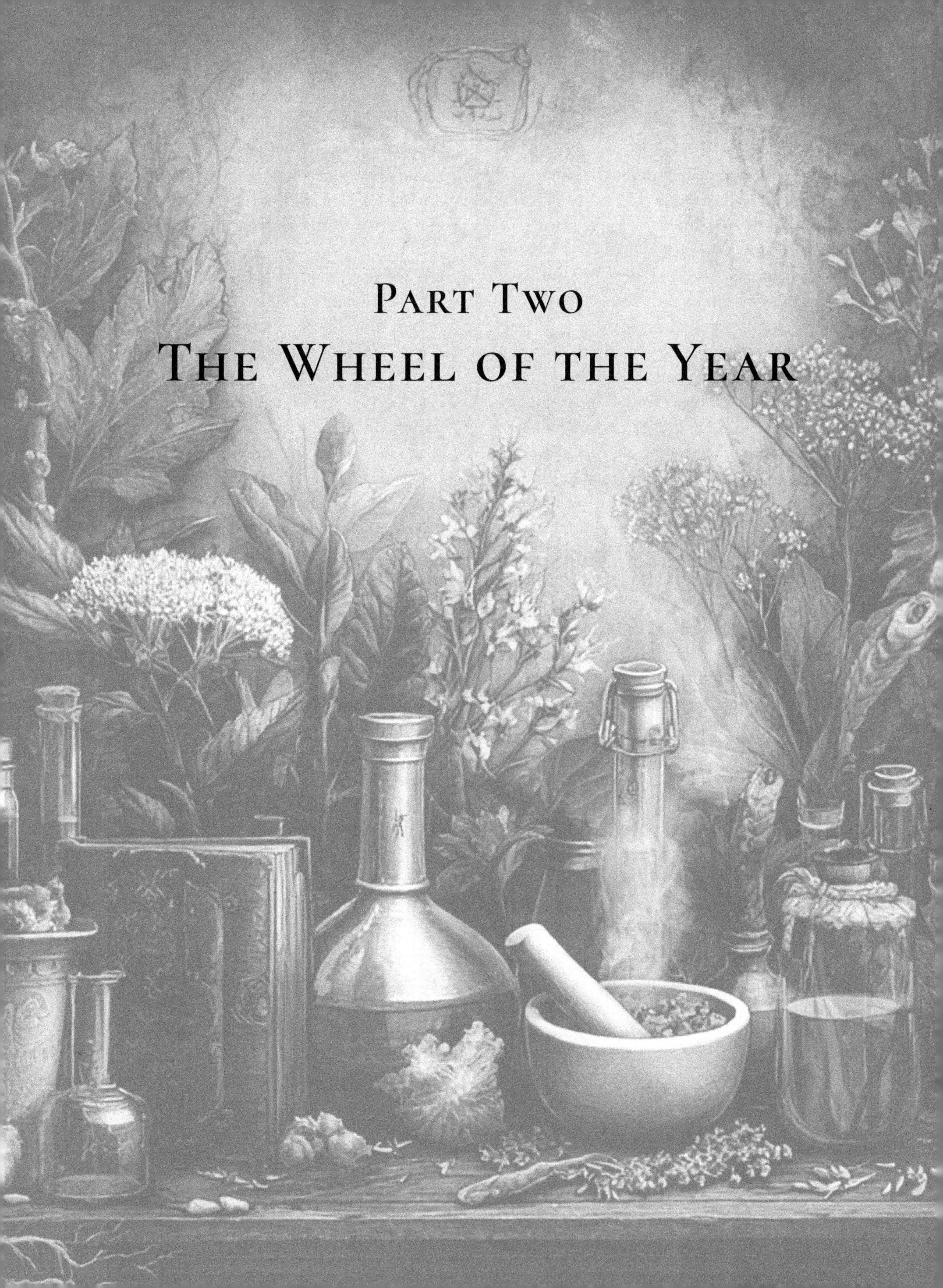

ON SEASONS

We speak of spring and summer, autumn and winter as if they were only calendar events - dates marked on a wall, weather patterns to dress for. **But the seasons are something far more fundamental!** They are patterns of energy that repeat at *every* scale of existence, from the cosmic to the cellular.

The year has its seasons, certainly. But so does a single day. Morning carries the energy of spring - emergence, awakening, the body rising from the dormancy of sleep into activity. Midday is summer - full expression, peak energy, the sun at its height. Afternoon moves into autumn - the beginning of descent, harvest, gathering what the day has produced. Night is winter - rest, withdrawal, conservation, the deep work that happens in darkness.

A human life moves through these same patterns. Childhood is spring - rapid growth, everything new, the body building itself toward fullness. Young adulthood is summer - peak vitality, outward expression, the full flowering of physical capacity. Middle age is autumn - the gathering of wisdom, the beginning of release, the shift from accumulation to discernment. Elder years are winter - conservation, inwardness, the deep knowing that comes from having lived through all the seasons before.

Even within illness and healing, the seasons turn. The acute phase of sickness is its own kind of winter - withdrawal, conservation, the body pulling resources inward to fight. Recovery is spring - the slow return of appetite, energy, engagement with the world. Full health is summer. And the wisdom gained from having been ill, the new awareness of what the body needs - that is autumn's harvest.

A woman's monthly cycle mirrors the year. Menstruation is winter - release, withdrawal, the shedding of what is no longer needed. The follicular phase is spring - building, rising energy, new possibilities. Ovulation is summer - full ripeness, peak fertility, maximum outward expression. The luteal phase is autumn - the gradual turning inward, the body preparing either for pregnancy or for release.

Why does this matter for herbalism?

Because understanding seasons as patterns rather than dates allows you to meet the body where it actually is. A person in the winter of their life has different needs than someone in summer - not just different herbs, but a different relationship to vitality, to rest, to what the body is asking for. A person whose constitution runs perpetually cold may need warming, summer-like support even in July. A person running hot may need cooling even in January.

The chapters that follow are organized around the wheel of the year - spring, summer, autumn, winter - because this is how our ancestors organized their relationship with plants, and because the literal seasons do shape what grows, what's available, and what the body tends to need. But as you read, remember that these patterns are fractal. They repeat at every scale. The wisdom of spring applies not just to March and April, but to morning, to childhood, to recovery, to any moment of emergence after dormancy.

Learn the seasons as energies, not just as dates. Then you can recognize them wherever they appear.

Chapter 5
Spring
Awakening and Cleansing

The Season of Rising

Spring is the season of emergence. What was dormant begins to stir. Seeds that waited through winter's cold swell with water and push upward toward light. Sap rises in trees, carrying stored sugars from root to branch. Birds return from wherever they wintered. The earth itself seems to exhale after holding its breath.

Your body knows this season, even if you spend your days indoors. You may feel the urge to clean, to clear, to organize - the nesting instinct turned outward. A natural desire to lighten your diet after winter's heavier fare. Increased energy and motivation, a restlessness that wasn't there in February. The need to move, to be outside, to feel sun on skin. A sense that something new is possible.

Spring's energy is upward and outward - the same direction sap moves, the same direction seeds grow. After winter's contraction, the body wants to expand. After months of conservation, it's ready to move what has been stored.

This is where the traditional concept of spring cleansing comes from - not as a punishing protocol or a wellness trend, but as a recognition that the body has natural rhythms of accumulation and release. Winter is for gathering and storing. Spring is for moving what has accumulated, lightening the load, preparing for summer's full expression.

But let's be clear about what we mean by cleansing. We're not talking about forcing the body through harsh protocols, aggressive fasting, or expensive supplements promising to flush toxins. The body already knows how to process and eliminate what it doesn't need - this is what the liver, kidneys, lymphatic system, skin, and colon do every moment of every day. What we're talking about is *supporting* these systems, creating conditions where they can work more efficiently, removing obstacles to their natural function.

The herbs and practices of spring support the body's own intelligence. They don't override it or force it. They work with the season's rising energy, helping the body do what it's already inclined to do.

THE DIGESTIVE SYSTEM: WHERE NOURISHMENT BEGINS

Digestion is where nourishment begins - and where many problems have their root. The digestive tract is a continuous tube from mouth to anus, some thirty feet of processing, absorbing, and eliminating. But it's far more than a tube.

Seventy percent of your immune system lives in the gut - the gut-associated lymphoid tissue that monitors everything passing through, distinguishing food from threat, friend from foe. A hundred million neurons line the digestive tract, forming what scientists now call the enteric nervous system, or "second brain" - capable of operating independently, communicating constantly with the brain in your head, influencing mood and cognition in ways we're only beginning to understand. Trillions of microbes make their home here, a community so vast and complex that it functions almost as an organ in itself, influencing everything from immune function to mental health to what foods you crave.

The gut is also a barrier - the boundary between the outside world (everything you swallow) and your inner world (the bloodstream, the tissues, the cells). When this barrier is compromised, substances that should stay in the gut leak into circulation, triggering immune responses that can manifest as inflammation anywhere in the body.

When digestion is working well, you know it mostly by absence - absence of complaint. Appetite is appropriate, neither excessive nor absent. Food digests without drama - no excessive gas, bloating, or discomfort. Bowel movements are regular, formed, and easy. Energy is sustained after eating rather than crashing. Skin is clear. Mind is clear.

When digestion struggles, the symptoms are hard to miss. Bloating, gas, cramping. Constipation or diarrhea, sometimes alternating unpredictably. Visible undigested food in stool. Fatigue after eating, as if the meal took more energy than it gave. Skin eruptions - acne, rashes, eczema - as the body tries to eliminate through the skin what the gut isn't handling. Brain fog, difficulty concentrating. Increasing food sensitivities, as the barrier becomes less discerning.

Many seemingly unrelated health issues trace back to the gut. Supporting digestive health is foundational - not because digestion is simple, but because it touches everything else.

THE LIVER: PROCESSING AND TRANSFORMATION

The liver is your body's great processor - a chemical factory performing over five hundred functions, most of them happening below conscious awareness. Everything absorbed from the digestive tract passes through the liver before reaching general circulation. This is the first line of processing: nutrients are sorted, stored, and distributed; potential toxins are identified and neutralized.

The liver handles the breakdown products of normal metabolism - the waste produced simply by being alive. It processes medications, alcohol, environmental chemicals, hormones that have done their work and need to be cleared. It converts fat-soluble compounds to water-soluble forms so they can be eliminated through urine or bile. This is not exotic detoxification - this is basic physiology, happening every moment in every human body.

Beyond processing, the liver is deeply involved in metabolism. It stores glucose as glycogen and releases it when blood sugar drops. It produces bile, which is essential for fat digestion and also a route of elimination. It synthesizes proteins, including those needed for blood clotting. It produces cholesterol - not the villain popular nutrition makes it out to be, but a necessary precursor for hormones, cell membranes, and vitamin D.

The liver also clears excess hormones from circulation. When liver function is sluggish, hormones that should be processed and eliminated can recirculate, creating imbalances. This is one reason why supporting liver function can help with hormonal issues - not because the liver produces hormones, but because it clears them.

How do you know if your liver is struggling under its load? Skin issues often appear - acne, unexplained rashes, itching without visible cause. Digestive difficulty with fatty foods, since bile production may be insufficient. Headaches, particularly frontal or behind the eyes. Poor tolerance for alcohol or rich foods - hangovers that seem disproportionate, heavy meals that sit like stones. For women, PMS and hormonal imbalances that seem resistant to other interventions.

Traditional systems often associated the liver with the emotions of frustration and anger - not because emotion originates in the liver, but because when liver energy is stuck, irritability often follows. Anyone who has felt the short temper that comes with a hangover knows this correlation directly.

The liver has remarkable regenerative capacity. It can regrow from as little as 25% of its original mass. Given adequate support and reduced burden, liver function often improves more readily than we might expect. The herbs of spring have traditionally supported this organ, and for good reason.

The Lymphatic System: The Slow River

If blood is the body's rushing river, lymph is its slow, quiet waterway - a parallel circulation that most people know little about. The lymphatic system drains excess fluid from tissues, preventing the swelling that would occur if all that fluid had nowhere to go. It transports immune cells throughout the body, providing surveillance and response. It filters out bacteria, viruses, and damaged cells through the lymph nodes - those small, bean-shaped organs that swell when you're fighting infection. It absorbs fats from the digestive system and returns proteins to the bloodstream.

Unlike blood, which is pumped by the heart, lymph has no central pump. It moves through muscle contraction, through deep breathing, through physical movement. When you're sedentary, lymph tends to stagnate. When you move, it flows. This is why exercise often leaves you feeling clearer, lighter - you've literally been pumping your lymphatic system.

Signs of lymphatic congestion include swollen lymph nodes, of course, but also more subtle patterns. Puffiness, especially in the morning or around the ankles and under the eyes. Breast tenderness, particularly premenstrually. Slow healing from cuts and infections. Frequent minor illnesses, as if the immune system isn't quite keeping up. A general sense of sluggishness, heaviness, feeling waterlogged.

Supporting lymphatic flow is essential for immune health and for helping the body clear what needs clearing. And unlike liver support, which is largely about herbs, lymphatic support is largely about movement. The herbs help, but the body moving through space is the primary pump.

The Skin: The Mirror and the Outlet

Your skin is both mirror and outlet. It reflects internal conditions - when digestion struggles, when liver is burdened, when lymph is stagnant, the skin often shows it. And it serves as an organ of elimination in its own right, releasing water-soluble wastes through sweat, fat-soluble compounds through sebum, and accumulated debris through the constant shedding of dead cells.

When the primary elimination pathways - liver, kidneys, colon - are overwhelmed, the skin takes on more of the burden. This is why liver congestion so often appears as acne, why constipation worsens eczema, why lymphatic stagnation shows as puffiness or that dimpled texture we call cellulite. The skin is doing what it can to help, excreting what other organs aren't managing to clear.

Supporting the skin means supporting all elimination pathways. When liver, lymph, kidneys, and colon are working well, the skin doesn't have to compensate. It can simply be skin - a boundary, a sensor, a regulator of temperature - rather than an overworked backup system.

Spring Support: The Gentle Approach

Modern wellness culture has made a commodity of cleansing - juice fasts that deplete protein, laxatives that damage intestinal flora, extreme restrictions that trigger rebound binging, expensive supplement protocols that promise to flush toxins as if the body were a clogged drain. This approach misunderstands the body's intelligence and often does more harm than good.

True spring support is gentle. It works with the body rather than against it. Support rather than force - your body knows how to process and eliminate; you're creating conditions that allow it to work more efficiently. Nourish rather than deprive - the liver needs protein and nutrients to do its processing work; starvation impairs rather than helps. Gradual rather than extreme - releasing stored compounds too quickly overwhelms the very systems meant to handle them. Seasonal rather than perpetual - spring support honors natural rhythms; it's not meant to be a year-round state of emergency.

What follows are the traditional tools for spring support - herbs and practices that have been used for generations to help the body do what spring invites it to do. Use them wisely, gently, in relationship with your own body's signals.

❧ Bitter Herbs: Waking the Digestive Fire

Bitter is the taste modern diets have largely eliminated - and the taste traditional medicine considered most essential. When bitter compounds touch the tongue, a cascade begins. Saliva production increases. The stomach begins secreting acid. The liver releases bile. The pancreas prepares enzymes. Peristalsis - the rhythmic contractions that move food through the tract - activates. All from a taste.

This bitter reflex improves virtually every aspect of digestion. Nutrients absorb better when stomach acid is adequate. Fats digest properly when bile flows. Elimination improves when peristalsis is strong. Blood sugar regulation improves when the pancreas is functioning well. All of this from remembering to taste bitter.

The key is that the bitter must be tasted - it's the taste receptors on the tongue that trigger the reflex. Bitter herbs in capsules, while they still have value, miss this initial activation. A few drops of bitter tincture on the tongue, a small sip of bitter tea, a salad of bitter greens - these engage the reflex fully.

Dandelion root and leaf are gentle bitters that also support liver function directly. Gentian is intensely bitter, a powerful digestive stimulant used in small amounts. Artichoke leaf is both bitter and liver-protective. Chamomile, often thought of as calming, is also a gentle bitter - its digestive benefits come partly from this quality. Yarrow combines bitterness with anti-inflammatory action.

Take bitters ten to fifteen minutes before meals. Just a small amount - a few drops of tincture, a small sip of strong tea. The goal is to taste the bitter, not to consume large quantities. This simple practice, done consistently, can transform digestion over time.

❧ Alterative Herbs: Gentle Clearing

Alteratives are what old herbals called "blood cleansers" - though the blood itself doesn't need cleansing so much as the systems that process it need support. These herbs work gently and gradually through multiple pathways: enhancing liver function, supporting kidney filtration, moving lymphatic fluid, encouraging elimination through the skin. They're not dramatic in their action - you won't feel them working the way you feel a laxative or a stimulant. But over weeks and months of consistent use, they shift the terrain.

Burdock root is perhaps the quintessential spring alterative - supporting liver processing, moving lymphatic stagnation, improving skin conditions from within. It's gentle enough for long-term use and can even be eaten as a vegetable, as it is in Japan under the name gobo. Burdock is a root, so you'll decoct it or use tincture.

Red clover blossoms support lymphatic clearing and are rich in minerals. They're mildly estrogenic, which makes them helpful for some hormonal patterns and contraindicated for others - know your situation before using. Infuse the dried flowers or use as tincture.

Cleavers is specific for lymphatic drainage - that sticky, clingy plant that grows wild in spring seems designed to help fluids move. It's cooling and drying, helpful where dampness and stagnation predominate. Cleavers is best used fresh - the fresh plant juice, a tea of the fresh plant, or a tincture made from fresh material. Dried cleavers loses much of its potency.

Nettles bridge the gap between alterative and nutritive - they support clearing while simultaneously nourishing with their rich mineral content. A long-steeped nettle infusion is both spring medicine and deep nourishment, particularly valuable when the body needs to clear without becoming depleted in the process.

❧ Liver-Supporting Herbs

Dandelion root is the friendliest liver herb - gentle, nourishing, safe for long-term use. It stimulates bile production, supports both phases of liver processing, and acts as a mild but effective bitter. You can drink it as a roasted root decoction, almost like a coffee substitute, or take it as tincture before meals. The whole plant is medicine - roots, leaves, and flowers each with their own gifts.

Milk thistle has become famous for liver protection, and for good reason. Its silymarin compounds have been extensively researched and shown to protect liver cells from damage and support regeneration. For anyone with a history of liver stress - from alcohol, medications, or environmental exposure - milk thistle offers real support. The seeds are typically used as tincture or standardized extract, as the compounds don't extract well into water.

Yellow dock root stimulates liver function and bile flow while also providing gentle laxative action - helpful when sluggish elimination is part of the pattern. It's also rich in iron, useful for building blood. Yellow dock is stronger than dandelion, more of a short-term intervention than a daily tonic.

❧ Lymphatic Support

Cleavers, mentioned above, is the premier lymphatic herb - use it freely in spring when it's growing fresh everywhere. Calendula, better known for wound healing, also moves lymphatic fluid and reduces inflammation. Red clover supports lymphatic clearing while nourishing with its mineral content.

But lymphatic support is primarily about movement. The lymphatic system has no pump of its own - it relies on muscle contraction, deep breathing, and physical activity to move its fluid. Daily walking supports lymph. Yoga, especially twists and inversions, helps lymph flow. Rebounding - gentle bouncing on a mini trampoline - is particularly effective because the rhythmic up-and-down motion helps the one-way valves in lymphatic vessels move fluid upward. Dry brushing the skin before showering stimulates superficial lymphatic flow while also exfoliating. Swimming, with its combination of movement and water pressure, provides excellent lymphatic support.

If you do nothing else for your lymphatic system, move your body daily. The herbs are helpers, but movement is the main medicine.

Eating With the Season

Spring eating naturally shifts toward the lighter, the fresher, the greener. After winter's heavier fare - the roots and meats and stored foods that sustained us through cold months - the body often craves exactly what spring provides: tender greens, bitter plants, the first fresh growth.

Bitter greens are spring's medicine in food form. Dandelion greens, arugula, endive, radicchio - these stimulate digestion and support liver function while providing nutrients. The bitter taste we've removed from modern diets is exactly what spring offers if we'll eat what's growing.

Cruciferous vegetables - broccoli, kale, cabbage, Brussels sprouts - contain compounds that support liver processing directly. These vegetables help the liver do its work more efficiently. They're available year-round now, but their traditional season began in spring with the early cabbages.

Fresh herbs - cilantro, parsley, dill, chives - begin appearing in spring gardens. These aren't just garnishes; they're concentrated plant medicine in culinary form. Use them liberally.

Spring is a natural time to reduce what burdens the liver: alcohol, heavily processed foods, excessive sugar, damaged fats. Not as punishment or deprivation, but as relief - giving the liver less to process so it can catch up on its backlog. This isn't about perfection or moral achievement. It's about creating space.

Adequate fiber matters more than most people realize. Fiber binds to bile in the intestines - bile that's carrying the compounds the liver has processed for elimination. Without adequate fiber, much of that bile gets reabsorbed and recycled, returning its load to the liver for reprocessing. Fiber ensures that what the liver has packaged for export actually leaves the body.

Hydration supports every elimination pathway. The kidneys need water to filter. The colon needs water to move waste. The skin needs water to sweat. There's no magic amount that applies to everyone - let thirst and the color of your urine guide you. Pale yellow suggests adequate hydration; dark yellow suggests you need more.

Living With the Season

Beyond herbs and food, spring asks for movement. The rising energy of the season wants to move through you, not stay stuck. Daily walking is perhaps the simplest and most accessible form - it supports digestion, lymphatic flow, mood, and circadian rhythm all at once. It asks nothing more than that you put one foot in front of the other.

Any movement you enjoy is good movement. Yoga, with its twists and folds, provides specific support for digestion and organ function. Dancing moves energy that might otherwise stagnate. Gardening - which begins in earnest in spring - combines movement with contact with soil and sun. The specific form matters less than the consistency and the enjoyment.

Sweating is elimination through the skin. Saunas, steam rooms, hot baths, or simply exercise that makes you sweat - all of these support the skin's eliminative function. If you have access to a sauna, spring is a traditional time to use it regularly. If not, hot baths with Epsom salts provide some of the same benefit while also delivering magnesium through the skin.

Rest remains important even as energy rises. The liver does much of its processing work at night during sleep. Going to bed earlier, sleeping more deeply, reducing the overscheduling that fragments rest - these support spring clearing as much as any herb. There's a temptation, as energy increases, to fill every moment with activity. Resist it. The rising energy needs rest to balance it.

Reducing your toxic load means less for the liver to process. This isn't about fear or purity; it's about simple arithmetic. Natural cleaning products, organic foods when possible (especially for the most heavily sprayed crops), filtered drinking water, personal care products without synthetic fragrances - these small choices add up over time, reducing the burden on systems already working hard.

When Spring Support Isn't Appropriate

Not everyone should emphasize clearing in spring. The body's wisdom doesn't always match the calendar.

Pregnancy and nursing are times for building, not clearing. The body is growing another human or producing milk; it needs its resources devoted to that work. Emphasize nourishment, not elimination.

If you're significantly underweight or malnourished, your body needs building, not lightening.

Spring support can be depleting for bodies that have nothing to spare. Focus on nourishing, grounding, substantive herbs and foods until your reserves are restored.

Active illness or infection is not the time to add the work of clearing. The body is already mobilized; let it fight. Support immunity, not elimination.

Recovery from surgery or major illness is a time for rebuilding. The body has been through trauma; it needs construction materials, not a push to release.

Those with a history of eating disorders should approach spring cleansing cautiously, if at all. The framework of cleansing can too easily feed into restrictive patterns. If this is your history, work with a practitioner who understands eating disorders, and emphasize nourishment over any form of restriction.

If you're already highly stressed or depleted - running on empty, exhausted, nothing left in reserve - more elimination will only deepen the hole. You need to build before you can afford to clear. Sometimes the most radical act is to rest and nourish rather than to cleanse.

Spring support should leave you feeling better - lighter, clearer, more energized. If you're feeling worse - more tired, more depleted, less well - that's information. Back off. Nourish. Trust your body's signals over any protocol, including this one.

Digestive Health Beyond Spring

While spring emphasizes clearing and lightening, digestive health matters year-round. Some fundamentals apply in every season.

Chew your food thoroughly. Digestion begins in the mouth, where enzymes in saliva start breaking down starches and mechanical chewing breaks food into smaller pieces. Swallowing half-chewed food forces the stomach to compensate. This is the simplest digestive intervention, and one of the most overlooked.

Avoid drinking large amounts of liquid with meals. Fluid dilutes stomach acid and digestive enzymes. Drink between meals instead, with just small sips during eating if needed. This simple change resolves digestive complaints for more people than you might expect.

Bitter herbs before meals - not just in spring, but year-round - support the entire digestive cascade. This is one of the most reliable interventions in herbal medicine, effective for a wide range of digestive complaints.

Eat mindfully. Put down the phone. Turn off the screen. Actually taste what you're eating. Notice when you're full. Stress shuts down digestion - the same nervous system that triggers fight-or-flight simultaneously suppresses digestive function. Eating in a calm state isn't precious advice; it's physiological necessity.

Regular mealtimes support digestion. The body prepares for meals when they come at predictable times, secreting digestive juices in anticipation. Erratic eating patterns mean the body is always caught off-guard.

Stop eating several hours before bed. Digestion slows at night as the body prepares for sleep. Late meals sit undigested, interfering with sleep quality and leaving you unrested. The traditional wisdom about not eating after dark has physiological basis.

EMBODIED PRACTICE: MAKING A SPRING BITTER FORMULA

This practice invites you into the kitchen to make actual medicine - a bitter tincture or tea blend that you'll use before meals throughout the spring season. This isn't a recipe to follow mechanically; it's a relationship to enter into. You'll meet the herbs, taste them, blend them according to your own intuition, and create something that's yours.

You'll need dried herbs - dandelion root, chamomile flowers, and dried ginger are a good starting place, though you can adapt based on what's available and what calls to you. You'll need either vodka for a tincture or just water for a tea blend. You'll need a jar for making tincture or a container for storing tea blend. And you'll need presence - the willingness to bring attention to the process, to taste and adjust, to make something rather than just follow instructions.

Read through the entire practice first. Then gather your materials and enter the kitchen as a place of alchemy.

❧ Gathering and Preparing

Clear your workspace. Bring out the herbs you'll be working with. You might use dandelion root and leaf for their liver support and gentle bitterness; chamomile for its calming bitter quality and ability to ease digestive tension; a small amount of ginger to warm the formula and activate the other herbs. These are suggestions, not requirements. Use what you have, what calls to you, what makes sense for your body.

Before you begin combining anything, meet each herb individually. Open each container. Smell deeply. Look at the color, texture, form. If the herb is safe to taste - and all the ones suggested here are - put a small pinch in your mouth and chew it slowly. What do you notice? What is its character? Its temperature? Its moisture? Let each herb introduce itself before you ask them to work together.

This is relationship, not just recipe-following. Take your time.

❧ If You're Making Tea Blend

For a tea blend, you're simply combining dried herbs in proportions that work for your palate and purpose. A suggested starting ratio: two parts dandelion root (roasted if you like a richer flavor, raw for more bitterness), one part chamomile flowers, and one-half part dried ginger. But taste as you go.

Combine a small amount first - perhaps a tablespoon total. Crush or crumble the herbs together with your fingers, letting them mingle. Bring water to a boil and make a test cup: put a teaspoon of your blend in a cup, pour hot water over, cover, and steep for ten minutes.

Taste your test cup. Is it bitter enough? Bitter should be present and clear, not overwhelming but not faint. If too mild, add more dandelion. Is it too bitter for you to actually drink it? Add more chamomile or ginger to soften. Is the ginger warmth right, or does it need more, or less? This is how you learn to formulate - by tasting, adjusting, tasting again.

When you're satisfied with the proportions, make a larger batch - perhaps a cup or two of dried blend, enough for several weeks of use. Store in a glass jar, labeled with the date and contents. Keep in a cool, dark place.

To use your bitter tea: steep one teaspoon per cup of water, covered, for ten to fifteen minutes. Drink a small cup - even just a few sips - ten to fifteen minutes before meals. The goal is to taste the bitter, not to consume large quantities.

❧ If You're Making Tincture

For a tincture, you'll be extracting the herbs into alcohol over several weeks. You'll need a clean glass jar - a pint mason jar works well - and vodka or brandy of at least 40% alcohol (80 proof).

Combine your dried herbs in the jar using proportions that feel right after your tasting. A suggested starting point: fill the jar one-quarter full with dandelion root, add chamomile to bring it to one-third full, then add a small amount of ginger - perhaps two tablespoons for a pint jar. But adjust based on your tasting and intuition.

Pour alcohol over the herbs until they're completely submerged, with at least two inches of liquid above them. Press down any floating herbs. All plant material must be below the surface or it will mold.

Label the jar immediately: what's in it, the proportions you used, the date, the type of alcohol. You will forget otherwise.

Cap tightly and place in a cool, dark location. Shake the jar daily - this is part of the practice, a daily moment of tending your medicine. Every time you shake it, you're in relationship with what you've made.

Let the tincture macerate for four to six weeks. Longer is stronger, but even two weeks will produce usable medicine if you're eager to begin.

When the time has come, strain through cheesecloth, squeezing the herbs to extract all the liquid. Bottle in amber glass, label again with contents and date. Store in a cool, dark place. Your tincture will remain potent for years.

To use your bitter tincture: take ten to thirty drops in a small amount of water ten to fifteen minutes before meals. Let it sit on your tongue for a moment - the bitter taste is part of how it works. Start with a smaller dose and increase if needed.

❧ The Ritual of Use

However you've made your bitter formula, the practice includes using it. Set it out where you'll see it before meals. Make taking your bitters a ritual - a moment of pause before eating, a way of signaling to your body that food is coming, a daily connection to the medicine you made with your own hands.

Notice what happens over days and weeks of consistent use. Does your appetite shift? Does digestion feel different? Does your energy after meals change? Keep notes if you like, or simply pay attention. You're building a relationship with these plants through daily use, learning how they work in your body.

At the end of spring - or whenever your formula runs out - you might make another batch, or you might be ready for something different. Let the seasons guide you. Let your body's responses guide you. The medicine you make is a living practice, evolving as you learn.

Reflection Questions

1. How is your digestion currently? What patterns do you notice - times of day, responses to certain foods, connection to stress?

2. Do you notice any signs that your liver is working hard - skin issues, difficulty with fats, irritability, headaches?

3. What does your lymphatic system tell you? Any puffiness, sluggishness, recurrent minor illnesses?

4. Which spring herbs call to you? When you taste them, what do you notice?

5. What dietary or lifestyle changes feel appropriate for you this season - not as rules, but as genuine invitations?

6. Where in your life are you in a "spring" phase - emerging, rising, moving from dormancy into expression? How might you support that transition?

Spring rises.
The body knows what this means.
Support the rising. Trust the body's intelligence. Let the clearing be gentle.

Chapter 6
Summer
Vitality and Protection

The Season of Full Expression

Summer is the culmination. Everything that emerged in spring, that pushed upward and outward with rising energy, now reaches its fullness. Days stretch to their longest. Warmth saturates the air. Plants flower and fruit. Life force is at its zenith - maximum expression, maximum activity, maximum connection with the world.

In your body, summer's energy manifests as capacity - the capacity for sustained activity, for being outdoors and in motion, for gathering with others, for projects that require full engagement. Circulation is strong, carrying oxygen and nutrients efficiently to every cell. The immune system is active, encountering more of the world as you move through it. There's an openness to summer, a permeability - windows open, skin exposed, the boundary between self and world more fluid than in winter's bundled containment.

But summer's gifts come with summer's demands. The same heat that ripens fruit can overheat a body. The same openness that allows connection also allows exposure - to sun, to allergens, to the microbes that travel when people gather. The abundance of activity can tip into depletion if you give more than you restore. Summer asks for protection even as it invites full expression.

This chapter explores the systems that keep you vital and protected during seasons of maximum output: the respiratory system, which exchanges your breath with the world; the immune system, which discerns friend from foe in everything you encounter; and the cardiovascular system, which circulates life through every part of you. These systems work hardest when you're most active, most exposed, most engaged with life. They deserve your attention and your care.

THE RESPIRATORY SYSTEM: THE BREATH BETWEEN WORLDS

Every breath is a conversation between your inner world and the outer world. You cannot survive more than a few minutes without this constant exchange - oxygen flowing in, carbon dioxide flowing out, the atmosphere entering your body and your body releasing into the atmosphere. Of all your body's relationships with the environment, breathing is the most intimate and the most continuous.

The respiratory tract begins with the nose and sinuses, which warm, filter, and humidify incoming air - preparing the outside world to meet your delicate lung tissue. Air travels down through the throat, past the vocal cords that give you voice, through the trachea that branches into bronchi, then into smaller and smaller bronchioles, finally reaching the alveoli - millions of tiny air sacs where the actual exchange happens. Oxygen crosses into blood; carbon dioxide crosses out. The whole system expands and contracts with each breath, twenty thousand times a day, mostly without your conscious attention.

The respiratory system is also your first line of defense against airborne threats. Mucus traps particles and pathogens; tiny hair-like cilia sweep debris upward and out; immune cells patrol the airways. When something harmful makes it past these defenses, inflammation, coughing, and increased mucus production mobilize to expel it. These responses feel unpleasant, but they are intelligent - your body doing exactly what it should.

Summer brings particular respiratory considerations. Pollen, mold, and grasses trigger allergic responses in sensitive airways. Travel and gatherings increase exposure to circulating viruses. Heat and exertion demand more oxygen, more breath, more work from a system already under seasonal pressure. And the very openness of summer - windows open, time spent outdoors - means the respiratory system encounters more of the world than it does in winter's relative isolation.

❧ When Breathing Becomes Struggle

Respiratory challenges range from the acute to the chronic, from the mild to the severe. The common cold - that familiar viral visitor - inflames the upper respiratory tract, producing congestion, runny nose, sore throat, and general misery. Influenza hits harder, with fever and body aches alongside respiratory symptoms. Bronchitis inflames the bronchi, producing a deep cough that may linger for weeks. Sinusitis congests the sinuses with pressure and pain. These acute conditions usually resolve, given time and support.

Chronic respiratory conditions require ongoing management. Asthma narrows and inflames the airways, producing wheezing, shortness of breath, and the frightening sensation of not being able to get enough air. Allergic rhinitis - hay fever - makes certain seasons miserable with congestion, itching, sneezing, and watery eyes. Chronic bronchitis keeps the bronchi perpetually inflamed. These conditions don't simply resolve; they require understanding, adaptation, and consistent support.

Understanding what your respiratory system needs in any given moment requires attention to what's actually happening. Is the cough productive, bringing up mucus that needs to leave? Or is it dry and hacking, irritating tissue without accomplishing anything? Is there heat and inflammation, or cold and stagnation? Are the airways constricted, or is the tissue simply irritated? These distinctions matter for choosing the right herbal support.

❧ How Herbs Support the Respiratory System

Different herbs work on the respiratory system in different ways. Understanding these actions helps you choose appropriately for the situation at hand.

Demulcent herbs soothe and coat irritated mucous membranes with their slippery, mucilaginous quality. When the cough is dry and hacking, when the throat is raw, when tissues are irritated and inflamed, demulcents bring relief. Marshmallow root, mullein, licorice, and slippery elm all offer this soothing, coating action.

Expectorant herbs help the body expel mucus from the respiratory tract. When congestion is sitting heavy in the lungs, when coughs are wet but unproductive, when mucus needs to move, expectorants assist its departure. Thyme, elecampane, horehound, and mullein all encourage expectoration, though through slightly different mechanisms - some by thinning mucus, others by stimulating the cough reflex, others by irritating the bronchi just enough to trigger clearing.

Antitussive herbs calm the cough reflex itself. This is appropriate when the cough is unproductive and exhausting - when nothing needs to come up but the coughing won't stop, especially at night when it prevents sleep. Wild cherry bark, licorice, and thyme all have antitussive properties. But be cautious with suppressing coughs - a productive cough that's moving mucus should generally be allowed to do its work, supported rather than silenced.

Antimicrobial herbs fight the infections that often underlie respiratory illness. Thyme, oregano, garlic, and eucalyptus all have demonstrated activity against bacteria, viruses, or both. These can be taken internally as teas or tinctures, or used as steam inhalations that deliver their volatile compounds directly to the airways.

Anticatarrhal herbs reduce excessive mucus production when the body is overproducing beyond what's needed. Goldenrod, elderflower, eyebright, and sage help moderate the flood when mucus has become more problem than solution.

Anti-allergic herbs reduce the histamine response that drives allergic symptoms. Nettles, eyebright, and goldenrod can help calm the overreaction of a system that's treating pollen as if it were a genuine threat.

Mullein: The Velvet Healer

Mullein is perhaps the quintessential respiratory herb - a tall, stately plant with velvety gray-green leaves that grows along roadsides and in disturbed places, offering its medicine freely to anyone who recognizes it. Its energetics are cool and moist, making it particularly suited for hot, dry, irritated respiratory conditions.

The leaves are demulcent and expectorant simultaneously - soothing irritated tissue while helping move stuck mucus. This makes mullein invaluable for dry, irritated coughs that nonetheless have congestion beneath; for bronchitis where expectoration is difficult; for any condition where the lungs feel both irritated and congested. It also has a relaxing quality that helps ease bronchial spasm, making it supportive for asthma alongside other interventions.

Mullein is also vulnerary - wound-healing - with an affinity for damaged lung tissue. Those recovering from pneumonia, from years of smoking, from any injury to the lungs find mullein's gentle repair support valuable.

The leaves are typically taken as infusion or tincture. One important note: mullein leaves are covered in fine hairs that can irritate the throat if not removed. Always strain mullein tea through a fine cloth or coffee filter, not just a regular strainer. The yellow flowers, infused in olive oil and allowed to steep in sunlight, make a traditional remedy for earaches - the oil warmed slightly and dropped into the affected ear.

Mullein is remarkably safe - gentle enough for children, appropriate for long-term use, with no significant contraindications. It's a plant you can befriend without worry.

Thyme: The Fierce Protector

Thyme brings a different energy to respiratory support - warm, dry, aromatic, actively antimicrobial. Where mullein soothes and repairs, thyme fights. Its volatile oils - particularly thymol and carvacrol - have demonstrated broad-spectrum activity against bacteria, viruses, and fungi. When infection is driving respiratory illness, thyme is an ally worth calling.

Thyme is both expectorant and antitussive, which might seem contradictory until you understand how it works. It helps thin and move mucus while also calming the spasmodic, unproductive coughing that exhausts without accomplishing anything. It's particularly valuable for productive coughs with infection - bronchitis, chest colds, the wet coughs that threaten to become something worse if not addressed.

The leaves and flowering tops are used, taken as tea, tincture, or honey infusion. For tea, covering while steeping is essential - those precious volatile oils will escape into the air if given the chance, carrying away much of the medicine. A steam inhalation with thyme brings its antimicrobial compounds directly to the airways - a bowl of steaming water, a handful of thyme, a towel over the head, breathing deeply for ten minutes.

Thyme is also a digestive antiseptic, helping clear gut infections and reduce harmful bacteria in the intestines. This makes it doubly valuable during illness, when both respiratory and digestive systems may be under assault.

Thyme is generally safe, though its essential oil can irritate skin if not properly diluted. For internal use, stick to the herb itself rather than the concentrated essential oil.

Elecampane: The Deep-Lung Mover

Elecampane is for the deep, stuck conditions - congestion that has settled into the lungs and refuses to move, chronic bronchitis that lingers month after month, lungs that feel perpetually heavy and wet. Its energetics are warm and slightly bitter, with an aromatic quality that penetrates into the depths of the respiratory tract.

The root is a powerful expectorant, helping dislodge and move mucus that has become entrenched. It's also warming and stimulating, making it particularly appropriate for cold, sluggish constitutional types and for conditions with a cold quality - pale mucus, cold chest, conditions that worsen in cold weather. For hot, inflammatory respiratory conditions, elecampane may be too warming; choose cooling alternatives instead.

Elecampane has a strengthening quality for weak lungs - lungs that catch every cold, that never quite recover from illness, that seem constitutionally vulnerable. Over time, elecampane can help build respiratory resilience in those who need it.

The root is decocted, tinctured, or made into syrup. Its flavor is distinctive - slightly bitter, aromatic, not unpleasant but clearly medicinal. Some people develop contact dermatitis from handling the fresh plant, so work with dried root if you're sensitive.

THE IMMUNE SYSTEM: DISCERNMENT AND DEFENSE

Your immune system is constantly asking questions: Self or other? Friend or foe? Safe or dangerous? Every moment, it monitors everything entering your body and everything arising within it, distinguishing what belongs from what doesn't, what can be tolerated from what must be eliminated. This is discernment on a cellular level - sophisticated, mostly invisible, absolutely essential.

The immune system is not a single organ but a network - a collaboration of barriers, cells, organs, and signaling molecules that together create your defense. Physical barriers form the first line: skin, mucous membranes, stomach acid, the beneficial bacteria that colonize your surfaces and compete with pathogens for resources. When something breaches these barriers, the innate immune response mobilizes - white blood cells that engulf invaders, inflammatory responses that wall off infection, fever that makes the body inhospitable to pathogens. This innate response is fast and non-specific; it attacks anything that seems like a threat.

The adaptive immune response is slower but more precise. T cells learn to recognize specific pathogens and destroy infected cells. B cells produce antibodies tailored to particular invaders. Memory cells remember what the body has encountered before, allowing faster response to repeat exposures. This is how vaccination works - introducing the immune system to a pathogen in a controlled way so it can remember and respond quickly if encountered again.

Seventy percent of your immune system lives in the gut - the gut-associated lymphoid tissue that monitors everything you swallow, distinguishing food from threat, helpful bacteria from harmful ones. This is why digestive health and immune health are so deeply intertwined. What you eat, the state of your microbiome, the integrity of your intestinal lining - all of this affects immune function directly.

❧ Two Ways of Working With Immunity

There are two fundamentally different approaches to supporting immunity with herbs, and understanding the distinction is crucial for appropriate use.

Immune stimulants activate the immune response - they sound the alarm, mobilize defenses, increase the activity and number of white blood cells fighting whatever has invaded. These herbs are powerful and appropriate *when you're actually fighting something* - at the first sign of a cold, during acute illness, when the immune system needs to mount a vigorous response. Echinacea, elderberry, and andrographis are immune stimulants.

But here's what's crucial: immune stimulants are for short-term use only. Days to two weeks at most. Using them continuously, month after month, exhausts the very system you're trying to support. It's like keeping soldiers on high alert indefinitely - eventually they collapse from the strain. People who take echinacea daily for "prevention" are misunderstanding how the herb works and may actually be weakening their immune response over time.

Immune stimulants are also generally inappropriate for autoimmune conditions, where the immune system is already overactive, attacking the body's own tissues. Stimulating an already hyperactive immune response makes autoimmune flares worse, not better.

Immune modulators work differently. Rather than stimulating the immune response, they help the immune system self-regulate - strengthening what's weak, calming what's overactive, building deep resilience over time. These herbs train the troops rather than mobilizing them for battle. Astragalus, reishi and other medicinal mushrooms, and adaptogenic herbs like holy basil and ashwagandha work as immune modulators.

Immune modulators are safe and appropriate for long-term use - months or years of daily consumption to build deep immunity. They're ideal for prevention during high-risk seasons, for recovery after illness when the immune system needs rebuilding, for anyone whose immunity seems chronically weak or dysregulated. They don't exhaust the system because they're not demanding action - they're building capacity.

Know which type you're using and why. Stimulants for acute illness, short-term. Modulators for building resilience, long-term. The distinction matters.

Elderberry: The Dark Medicine

Elderberry has become deservedly famous as an immune-supporting herb, particularly for preventing and shortening influenza. Research has shown that elderberry compounds interfere with the virus's ability to enter cells and replicate, and that people who take elderberry at the onset of flu recover faster than those who don't. This isn't folk medicine wishful thinking - it's been demonstrated in clinical trials.

The dark purple-black berries are rich in anthocyanins - the same antioxidant compounds that make blueberries and blackberries valuable - along with vitamin C and various flavonoids that support immune function. The berries are cooling and moistening, appropriate for hot, feverish conditions.

Elderflowers - the creamy white blossoms that precede the berries - have their own gifts. They're diaphoretic, meaning they promote sweating, making them valuable for breaking fevers and supporting the body's natural fever process. Elderflower tea is a traditional remedy for the early stages of colds and flu, especially when fever is present.

One critical safety note: raw elderberries, as well as the leaves, stems, and bark, contain cyanogenic glycosides - compounds that release cyanide in the body. *Raw elderberries must never be consumed.*

Cooking destroys these compounds completely, making the prepared berries entirely safe. Elderberry syrup, properly made with cooked berries, is safe for children and adults alike. But never eat raw elderberries, and never prepare medicine from the leaves, stems, or bark.

Elderberry is an immune stimulant, not a modulator, which means it should be used for prevention during active exposure or for treatment during illness - not taken daily for months on end. During cold and flu season, many people take elderberry syrup daily as a preventive when they know they'll be exposed (travel, gatherings, work with the public). During active illness, it can be taken every few hours. But in the off-season, let it rest.

Echinacea: The Quick Responder

Echinacea is probably the most well-known immune herb in North America, and for good reason - when used correctly, it's remarkably effective at supporting the body's response to early infection. The key words there are "used correctly." Echinacea is widely misused, taken in ways that don't work or that actually undermine immune function over time.

Echinacea works as an immune stimulant, increasing white blood cell activity and enhancing phagocytosis - the process by which immune cells engulf and destroy pathogens. It also has antimicrobial and anti-inflammatory properties, and supports lymphatic movement. The fresh root is generally considered most potent, particularly from Echinacea angustifolia, though E. purpurea is more commonly available and still effective.

Here's how to use echinacea effectively: at the *very first sign* of infection - that scratchy throat, that first sneeze, that vague sense that something is coming on - take echinacea tincture intensively. This means substantial doses every two hours for the first day or two, not a few drops once a day. Some herbalists recommend as much as a teaspoon of tincture every two hours initially. Then taper to three or four times daily as symptoms improve. Continue for a few days after you feel better, then stop.

The whole treatment might last a week. Then you're done until the next infection threatens. Taking echinacea continuously "for prevention" doesn't prevent anything - it exhausts immune response over time. Taking tiny doses once a day during illness doesn't do much either. Echinacea needs to be used intensively and briefly to work.

Quality matters enormously with echinacea. The market is flooded with low-quality products that don't contain what they claim. Good echinacea tincture produces a distinctive tingling sensation on the tongue - if you don't feel that tingle, the product may not be effective. Source from reputable suppliers who can verify the identity and potency of their material.

Echinacea should be avoided by those with autoimmune conditions, as stimulating an already overactive immune system is counterproductive. Those with Asteraceae allergies (ragweed, chamomile, etc.) occasionally react to echinacea, though this is less common than sometimes suggested.

Astragalus: The Deep Builder

Astragalus represents a completely different approach to immune support - the slow, steady building of deep resilience rather than the acute mobilization of defenses. This is an immune modulator, safe and appropriate for months of continuous use, gradually strengthening the body's capacity to defend itself.

The root is warming and sweet, building vital energy over time. It increases the production of immune cells, enhances their activity, and helps the body self-regulate rather than simply ramp up response. It's also adaptogenic, supporting the stress response alongside immunity - valuable because chronic stress is one of the most reliable immune suppressors.

Astragalus is traditionally used for those who catch every cold, whose recovery from illness is slow, whose immunity seems constitutionally weak. It's taken during the recovery phase after acute illness to rebuild what was spent. It's taken throughout cold and flu season to build resilience. It's taken by those undergoing chemotherapy or radiation (under practitioner supervision) to protect and restore immune function.

The traditional way to use astragalus is to add the dried root slices to soups and broths - it simmers for hours, releasing its medicine into the liquid, the spent roots discarded before eating. This makes immune support a part of nourishment rather than a separate supplement to remember. Astragalus can also be decocted as tea or taken as tincture.

Traditional use avoids astragalus during acute infection - the thinking being that you don't want to modulate the immune response while it's actively fighting; you want it to fight unimpeded. Use astragalus before illness to build resistance, or after illness to recover - but switch to acute-phase herbs like echinacea or elderberry during active infection.

The Cardiovascular System: The Tireless River

Your heart beats approximately one hundred thousand times every day. It began beating before you were born and will continue until you die, never once stopping to rest. This fist-sized muscle pumps two thousand gallons of blood through sixty thousand miles of blood vessels daily - arteries carrying oxygen-rich blood outward, capillaries exchanging nutrients and waste at the cellular level, veins returning oxygen-depleted blood for renewal. The whole system forms a continuous circuit, a river that flows in one direction, endlessly.

The heart itself is both simple and sophisticated. Four chambers - two atria receiving blood, two ventricles pumping it out. Valves ensuring one-way flow. An electrical conduction system that coordinates each beat, setting the rhythm without any conscious input. Coronary arteries feeding the heart muscle itself, because even the pump needs nourishment. When any of these components fails or falters, the consequences ripple through every cell that depends on circulation for life.

What the cardiovascular system delivers is life itself - oxygen to fuel cellular metabolism, nutrients to build and repair, hormones carrying messages, immune cells on patrol, heat distributed to maintain temperature. What it removes is waste - carbon dioxide, metabolic byproducts, cellular debris. Every cell in your body depends on this delivery and removal system working continuously. The brain, which is only two percent of body weight but consumes twenty percent of circulating oxygen, is exquisitely sensitive to any interruption in flow.

Summer places particular demands on the cardiovascular system. Heat dilates blood vessels, requiring the heart to work harder to maintain blood pressure. Sweating depletes fluids and electrolytes. Increased activity demands increased oxygen delivery. For those with cardiovascular vulnerability, summer's heat can be genuinely dangerous. For everyone, summer asks that we attend to what keeps circulation strong and the heart well-nourished.

❧ The Heart's Needs

Cardiovascular health depends on a web of factors - some within our control, some less so. Family history matters; some people are genetically more vulnerable. But lifestyle choices matter more than most people realize.

Movement is perhaps the heart's most essential medicine. The heart is a muscle, and like all muscles, it grows stronger with appropriate challenge. Regular moderate exercise - walking, swimming, cycling, dancing, anything that raises the heart rate for sustâined periods - builds cardiovascular capacity over time. Sedentary living, conversely, allows the heart to weaken, the vessels to stiffen, the whole system to become less resilient.

What you eat shapes cardiovascular health profoundly. Diets rich in vegetables, fruits, whole grains, fish, and healthy fats - what's sometimes called a Mediterranean pattern - consistently show protective effects. Diets heavy in processed foods, sugar, and damaged fats promote inflammation and arterial damage. The vessel walls are living tissue, constantly being damaged and repaired; what you eat determines whether that repair process keeps up with the damage.

Chronic stress is a cardiovascular stressor. The stress response raises blood pressure, increases heart rate, promotes inflammation, and over time contributes to arterial damage. Learning to manage stress - through movement, breath work, meditation, connection, enjoyable activities, whatever works for you - is cardiovascular medicine as much as any herb.

Sleep matters more than most people appreciate. During sleep, the cardiovascular system gets its only real rest - heart rate drops, blood pressure falls, repair processes activate. Chronic sleep deprivation is a cardiovascular risk factor independent of everything else. The heart cannot run at full capacity indefinitely; it needs its nightly recovery.

Smoking is perhaps the most damaging thing you can do to your cardiovascular system - every cigarette causes measurable arterial damage. This is not a case for moderation; there is no safe level. If cardiovascular health matters to you, tobacco has to go.

Hawthorn: Heart Medicine

Hawthorn is the great heart herb of the Western tradition - a thorny tree that has been used for centuries to strengthen and protect the cardiovascular system. Its berries, leaves, and flowers all carry medicine, and it's one of the few herbs with enough research behind it that even conventional medicine acknowledges its value.

Hawthorn works on the heart in several ways. It strengthens the heart muscle's contractions - the technical term is positive inotropic effect - allowing the heart to pump more efficiently. It dilates the coronary arteries, improving blood flow to the heart muscle itself. It protects blood vessels with its rich antioxidant content, particularly the flavonoids and oligomeric proanthocyanidins (OPCs) that give the berries their deep red color. It has a mild blood pressure lowering effect, making it supportive for those with hypertension.

What's remarkable about hawthorn is its normalizing quality. It's not simply stimulating or sedating to the heart - it helps the heart find its appropriate rhythm, whatever that is. People with high blood pressure find it helps lower. People with low blood pressure sometimes find it helps raise. People with irregular heartbeat often find it helps regulate. This balancing quality is uncommon and valuable.

Hawthorn's effects are gradual - this is not a rescue remedy for acute cardiac events. It builds over weeks and months of consistent use, slowly strengthening and protecting. This makes it ideal for long-term cardiovascular support, and it's safe enough for exactly that purpose. Many people take hawthorn daily for years as heart nourishment.

The berries are traditionally decocted; the leaves and flowers infused. Tincture works well. Some people make a hawthorn elixir with honey and brandy, combining the berries' medicine with the preserving and extracting power of alcohol and the nourishment of honey.

There's also an emotional dimension to hawthorn's medicine. Traditionally, it's associated with the grieving heart, the heart that has been wounded by loss or disappointment. Those going through heartbreak, processing grief, or recovering from emotional trauma find hawthorn supportive in ways that go beyond physical cardiovascular function. The heart, after all, is more than a pump.

Hawthorn is very safe, even alongside cardiac medications - though if you're on heart drugs, keep your healthcare provider informed, as hawthorn may enhance their effects over time. It's not a replacement for emergency cardiac care; chest pain, severe shortness of breath, signs of heart attack or stroke require immediate medical attention.

Garlic: The Pungent Protector

Garlic is food and medicine simultaneously - one of those plants so deeply woven into human culture that we forget it's medicinal at all. But the cardiovascular benefits of regular garlic consumption are well-documented, making this humble kitchen staple a genuine heart ally.

Garlic's cardiovascular gifts come largely from allicin, a sulfur compound formed when garlic is crushed or chopped - the same compound responsible for garlic's pungent smell. Allicin relaxes blood vessel walls, helping lower blood pressure. It interferes with cholesterol synthesis in the liver, helping reduce circulating cholesterol levels. It has antiplatelet effects, making blood less likely to form dangerous clots. And it's antimicrobial, fighting infections throughout the body.

To maximize garlic's medicinal value, crush or chop it and let it sit for ten minutes before cooking or eating. This waiting period allows the enzymatic reaction that produces allicin to complete. Cooking immediately after cutting destroys the enzyme before it can do its work. Heat also degrades allicin, so while cooked garlic still has value, raw garlic is more medicinally potent.

One or two raw cloves daily provides cardiovascular support. Some people mince a clove into honey, which both preserves the garlic and makes it more palatable. Others add raw garlic to salad dressings, pestos, or guacamole just before eating. Still others simply accept the intensity and chew a clove followed by parsley or mint to soften the breath. Aged garlic extract, available commercially, provides benefits with less of the pungency.

Garlic's antiplatelet effect means it should be discontinued before surgery and used cautiously by those on blood-thinning medications - the effects can compound. It can cause heartburn in sensitive individuals. And yes, there is the social consideration of garlic breath and body odor, which some consider a fair price for the medicine and others find prohibitive. Parsley, chlorophyll, and mint help, but nothing eliminates it entirely.

When to Seek Medical Care

Herbs support cardiovascular health beautifully, but they work alongside medical care, not instead of it. Know when the situation calls for professional intervention.

Some situations are emergencies. Chest pain, pressure, or discomfort - especially if it spreads to the arm, jaw, or back - requires immediate medical attention. Severe shortness of breath that comes on suddenly. Signs of stroke: facial drooping, arm weakness, speech difficulty. Sudden severe headache unlike any you've had before. Loss of consciousness. Severe allergic reaction with throat swelling or difficulty breathing. These are situations where minutes matter; call emergency services immediately.

Other situations warrant medical evaluation without the same urgency. Consistently elevated blood pressure - readings repeatedly above 140/90 - needs assessment and monitoring. Palpitations or irregular heartbeat that persists or recurs. Shortness of breath with exertion that's new or worsening. Swelling in the legs or ankles that doesn't resolve. A strong family history of heart disease, which means you should be screened earlier and more carefully. Any cardiovascular symptoms that concern you - trust that concern and get evaluated.

Respiratory situations also sometimes need medical care. Difficulty breathing that's severe or worsening. Fever that's very high or that doesn't respond to supportive measures. Respiratory infection that isn't improving after a week, or that's getting worse. Coughing up blood. Wheezing or asthma that's not responding to your usual interventions. When in doubt, get checked.

The herbs in this chapter support the systems that keep you vital and protected. They are not substitutes for medical care when medical care is needed. Know the difference. Trust your judgment. Seek help when the situation calls for it.

EMBODIED PRACTICE: MAKING A HAWTHORN HEART ELIXIR

This practice invites you to make a traditional heart elixir - hawthorn berries extracted into honey and brandy, creating a medicine that nourishes the cardiovascular system while being genuinely pleasurable to take. An elixir combines the extractive power of alcohol with the preserving and sweetening qualities of honey, making medicine that's both effective and delicious.

You'll need dried hawthorn berries - available from herbal suppliers or wild-harvested if you have access to hawthorn trees and can identify them confidently. You'll need raw honey, preferably local. You'll need brandy or another spirit of at least 40% alcohol. You'll need a clean glass jar with a tight-fitting lid. And you'll need patience - this elixir takes several weeks to make and then rewards you for months or years.

Read through the entire practice first. Then gather your materials and enter the kitchen as a place of alchemy.

❧ Gathering and Preparing

Clear your workspace. Set out your hawthorn berries, honey, brandy, and jar. Take a moment to consider what you're about to make - medicine for the heart, both physical and emotional. Let that intention settle into your body.

If your hawthorn berries are whole, you can use them as-is or gently crush them to expose more surface area for extraction. Crushing isn't essential but speeds the process slightly. You can crush them with a mortar and pestle, roll them with a rolling pin, or pulse briefly in a blender.

Before you begin combining, take a moment with the hawthorn. Smell the dried berries - they have a subtle, slightly sweet, almost apple-like aroma. If you like, taste one - they're safe to eat, mildly sweet and astringent. This is the plant you're inviting into relationship with your heart.

❧ Combining

Fill your jar about one-third full with hawthorn berries. Don't pack them too tightly - they need room for liquid to circulate.

Now add honey until the jar is about half full. The honey will be thick and slow - let it settle down around the berries, coating them. You can warm the honey gently (not hot - that damages its beneficial properties) to make it flow more easily if it's very solid.

Pour brandy over the honey and berries until the jar is nearly full, leaving about an inch of headspace. The brandy will be lighter than the honey and will float on top initially. That's fine - you'll be mixing it.

Cap the jar tightly and shake well, turning it upside down and back several times. Your goal is to blend the honey and brandy together around the berries. The honey will dissolve slowly into the brandy over time, but shaking accelerates the process.

Label the jar clearly: Hawthorn Heart Elixir, the date, and what's in it. This label will matter in a few weeks when you've forgotten exactly when you made it.

❧ The Waiting and Tending

Place your jar in a cool, dark location - a cupboard, a closet, somewhere out of direct light. Light degrades both herbs and honey over time.

For the next four to six weeks, shake the jar daily. This is part of the practice - a daily moment of tending your medicine, a daily reminder of what you're creating for your heart. Turn it upside down, right side up, swirl it around. The honey will gradually dissolve completely into the brandy, and the berries will release their medicine into the menstruum.

You'll notice the color deepening as the weeks pass - the liquid taking on a rich, reddish-amber hue as the hawthorn's compounds extract. This is visible alchemy, the transformation happening before your eyes.

❧ Straining and Bottling

After four to six weeks - or longer if you prefer; more time extracts more medicine - strain your elixir through cheesecloth or a fine-mesh strainer. Squeeze the berries to extract all the precious liquid they've absorbed.

Bottle the strained elixir in clean glass jars or amber bottles. Label again with contents and date. Stored in a cool, dark place, your elixir will remain potent for years - the alcohol and honey together create an exceptionally stable preparation.

The spent hawthorn berries can go to compost, their medicine now transferred to your elixir.

❧ The Ritual of Use

To use your hawthorn elixir, take one to two teaspoons daily, either straight or in a small amount of water. Some people take it first thing in the morning as a heart tonic to start the day. Others take it in the evening as a gentle unwinding, the brandy adding a relaxing quality. Find the rhythm that works for you.

The effects of hawthorn are gradual - you won't feel a dramatic shift immediately. Over weeks and months of consistent use, you may notice your cardiovascular system functioning more smoothly, your blood pressure more stable, your heart feeling generally stronger. Or you may simply have the quiet knowledge that you're nourishing this vital organ daily.

This is also medicine for the emotional heart. During times of grief, heartbreak, or emotional strain, hawthorn elixir offers gentle support. The heart that has been wounded - by loss, by disappointment, by life's inevitable sorrows - finds solace in hawthorn's medicine.

❧ Variations

Once you've made the basic hawthorn elixir, you might explore variations. Some people add rose petals, bringing in rose's own heart-opening and emotionally soothing qualities. A few slices of fresh ginger add warmth, supporting circulation. A cinnamon stick brings its own cardiovascular benefits along with warming sweetness. Hibiscus flowers, which have their own mild blood pressure lowering effect, add a beautiful red color and tart flavor.

Each addition changes the medicine slightly. Let your intuition and your heart's needs guide what you include. There's no wrong way to make this elixir - only your way, which you'll refine over time as you learn what your heart asks for.

Reflection Questions

1. How is your respiratory health? Do you notice patterns - seasonal allergies, frequent colds, sensitivity to air quality?

2. What is your relationship with your immune system? Does it feel robust and balanced, or does it seem to need support? In what direction - more strength, or more regulation?

3. How does your heart feel - physically and emotionally? What does your cardiovascular system need?

4. Which summer herbs call to you? When you read about them, which ones resonate?

5. What practices - beyond herbs - might support your vitality and protection? Movement, rest, stress management, connection?

6. Where in your life are you in a "summer" phase - full expression, maximum output, the peak of a cycle? How might you protect your radiance even as you share it?

Summer offers its fullness.
Protect the systems that allow you to shine.
Care for your breath, your defenses, your tireless heart.

Chapter 7
Autumn
Gathering and Grounding

The Season of Consolidation

Autumn is the great gathering. What was scattered outward through summer's expansive heat now begins its return - leaves falling, sap descending, seeds dropping to earth. The energy that rose and bloomed and fruited is consolidating, preparing, storing. There's a turning inward that you can feel in the air itself, a quality of descent and collection.

Your body mirrors this gathering, whether you consciously recognize it or not. You may feel the urge to organize, to prepare, to nest - clearing out what's no longer needed, making space for what matters. Appetite often increases as the body intuitively seeks to build reserves for the darker months ahead. Sleep needs lengthen as the days shorten, the body asking for more rest even as the culture insists on maintaining summer's pace. There's a natural desire to slow down, to turn attention from the external world to the internal one, to shift focus from expansion to foundation.

Autumn invites you to resource yourself - not in the superficial sense of self-care products and weekend retreats, but in the deeper sense of actually building the reserves that will sustain you through winter's demands. This means nourishing your nervous system, which has likely been running on overdrive through summer's activity. It means strengthening your bones and structure, the literal foundation that holds you upright. It means gathering what you need before the season of scarcity arrives.

This chapter explores the systems of communication and structure: the nervous system, your body's vast electrical network that coordinates everything you think, feel, and do; and the skeletal system, the mineral-rich framework that gives you form. Both require nourishment. Both benefit from autumn's gathering energy. Both will serve you better through winter if you attend to them now.

THE NERVOUS SYSTEM: THE BODY'S ELECTRICAL WEB

Your nervous system is vast beyond easy comprehension - billions of neurons connected by trillions of synapses, forming a communication network that makes the internet look simple. It's the command center that processes every sensation and generates every response. It's the electrical web that coordinates every movement, conscious and unconscious. It's the substrate of thought, emotion, memory, personality - everything that makes you recognizably you.

The central nervous system - brain and spinal cord - forms the core, processing information and issuing commands. The peripheral nervous system branches outward to every corner of the body, carrying sensory information in and motor commands out. Within the peripheral system, the somatic nerves handle voluntary movement and conscious sensation, while the autonomic nerves manage the involuntary functions - heartbeat, digestion, breathing, all the processes that continue whether you think about them or not.

The autonomic nervous system deserves particular attention, because it's where most modern people run into trouble. It has two branches: the sympathetic, which activates the stress response - fight, flight, freeze - and the parasympathetic, which governs rest, digestion, and healing. These two branches are meant to balance each other, the sympathetic mobilizing resources for threat, the parasympathetic allowing recovery when the threat has passed.

There's also the enteric nervous system - the "second brain" embedded in the walls of your digestive tract. A hundred million neurons live there, producing neurotransmitters including roughly ninety percent of the body's serotonin. This gut-brain communicates constantly with the head-brain through the vagus nerve, which is why emotional states affect digestion and digestive states affect mood. You've felt this if you've ever had butterflies in your stomach before a stressful event, or felt anxious when your digestion was off.

❧ The Modern Nervous System Crisis

Modern life keeps most people in chronic sympathetic activation - the stress response running continuously, never fully switching off to allow parasympathetic recovery. This isn't how the system was designed to work. The sympathetic response evolved for acute threats - the predator, the rival, the sudden danger that required immediate action. It was meant to activate intensely and briefly, then resolve completely as the parasympathetic took over for rest and repair.

Instead, we face chronic, unresolvable stressors - work pressures that never end, financial anxieties that persist for years, relationships that remain difficult, news cycles that deliver fresh threats hourly. The sympathetic system activates but has no clear signal that the danger has passed, so it stays activated. Meanwhile, we undermine parasympathetic function through poor sleep, constant stimulation, irregular schedules, and caffeine dependence that keeps us artificially alert when the body is asking for rest.

The results are familiar to almost everyone. Anxiety and restlessness that seem to have no specific cause. Insomnia - difficulty falling asleep, staying asleep, or waking rested. Difficulty concentrating, the scattered thinking that gets labeled brain fog. The exhaustion that coexists with inability to relax, the "wired but tired" pattern that signals a nervous system running on empty while refusing to stop. Physical tension that accumulates in the jaw, the shoulders, the back. Digestive issues that resist dietary interventions because the problem isn't what you're eating but the state you're in while eating it. Weakened immunity, because chronic stress suppresses immune function. Depression, as neurotransmitter reserves deplete and the capacity for joy erodes.

This is the nervous system crisis of our time. It's not a personal failing; it's a mismatch between how we're living and how we're built. And it requires more than a vacation or a good night's sleep to address - though those help. It requires systematic nourishment and rebuilding of a system that has been depleted by demands it was never designed to handle.

THREE WAYS HERBS SUPPORT THE NERVOUS SYSTEM

Herbs that support the nervous system - collectively called nervines - work in different ways. Understanding these categories helps you choose appropriately for what you actually need, which may be different from what you think you need.

❧ Nervine Relaxants: Releasing the Grip

Nervine relaxants calm an overactive nervous system in the moment. They reduce tension and anxiety, promote relaxation, help quiet the racing mind. Their effects are relatively quick - minutes to hours - making them valuable for acute situations. When you can't fall asleep because your mind won't stop, when anxiety is spiking before a difficult conversation, when accumulated tension has your shoulders up around your ears, nervine relaxants can help.

Chamomile is the gentlest of the relaxants, safe for children and elders, mild enough for daily use yet effective for genuine anxiety. Lemon balm combines nervine relaxation with an uplifting quality that prevents the heaviness some people feel with sedating herbs, and it supports digestion simultaneously - valuable when stress has disrupted the gut. Passionflower is stronger, a genuine anxiolytic and sleep aid that works on GABA pathways similarly to pharmaceutical anti-anxiety drugs but more gently. Valerian is powerful sedation, not subtle at all, useful when you need to simply knock out the stress response and sleep. Skullcap specifically calms the racing, circular thoughts that keep many people awake. Lavender brings its aromatic medicine, helpful particularly for tension headaches and anxiety with a physical tension component.

Nervine relaxants can be used as needed for acute situations, or taken regularly during particularly stressful periods. They're not building anything - they're releasing what's gripped. That's valuable, but it's not the whole picture.

❧ Nervine Tonics: Rebuilding the Foundation

Nervine tonics work differently. Rather than releasing tension in the moment, they nourish and rebuild the nervous system over time. They restore depleted reserves. They strengthen the system's resilience so that it can handle stress without being overwhelmed. Their effects are not immediate -

they work slowly over weeks and months of consistent use. But they address the root problem rather than just managing symptoms.

These are the herbs for burnout, for exhaustion, for nervous systems that have been running on empty for so long they've forgotten what resourced feels like. For recovery from prolonged stress or trauma. For building the kind of deep resilience that means you can face challenges without being shattered by them.

Milky oat tops is perhaps the supreme nervine tonic - deeply nourishing, restorative in a way that feeds the nervous system at its root. Skullcap, unusually, works as both relaxant and tonic, providing immediate relief while building long-term strength. St. John's wort supports mood and helps with nerve pain, rebuilding what depression has depleted. Gotu kola supports cognitive function and may actually help regenerate nerve tissue. Wood betony grounds and clears mental fog, bringing scattered energy back to center.

Nervine tonics require patience. Minimum six weeks of consistent use, often twelve weeks or more, to see their full effects. This is not a quick fix; it's a rebuilding project. But for those whose nervous systems are genuinely depleted, quick fixes don't actually fix anything. Only nourishment over time can restore what has been exhausted.

❧ Nervine Stimulants: A Word of Caution

Nervine stimulants increase alertness, improve focus, provide mental energy. Rosemary, peppermint, green tea, coffee - these are the herbs that wake things up, sharpen attention, get you going when fatigue threatens to stop you.

Here's the caution: most modern people need *less* stimulation, not more. The nervous systems around us are not sluggish; they're exhausted. They're already running on adrenaline and cortisol and caffeine. Adding more stimulation to an exhausted system doesn't restore it - it depletes it further. It's like whipping a tired horse; you might get a burst of speed, but you're damaging the animal.

If you're relying on stimulants to function - needing coffee to wake up, needing more coffee to stay focused, crashing when the caffeine wears off - that's information about the state of your nervous system. The answer isn't more stimulants; it's addressing the root cause. Better sleep. Better nutrition. Less chronic stress. More parasympathetic time. Nervine tonics to rebuild what's been depleted.

There's a place for stimulants - used sparingly, for temporary situations when alertness genuinely matters. But they should be the exception, not the daily crutch. If they've become essential to your functioning, that's a signal to attend to your nervous system's actual needs.

Meeting the Nervine Herbs

Milky Oat Tops: The Deep Nourisher

Milky oat tops come from the common oat plant, but harvested at a very specific moment - when the seed heads are still green and, if you squeeze them, exude a white, milky liquid. This brief window, lasting only about a week, is when the plant contains maximum nervine constituents. Miss the window and you have oatstraw, still valuable for minerals, but lacking the profound nervine potency of the milky stage.

The medicine of milky oats is deep nourishment for the nervous system - not stimulation, not sedation, but actual feeding of depleted nerve tissue. Its energetics are neutral, sweet, moist - the qualities of true nourishment. It rebuilds what has been exhausted, restores the capacity to feel without being overwhelmed, supports the nervous system in recovering its natural resilience.

Milky oats is specific for the frazzled, depleted person - the one who has been running on stress hormones for so long they've forgotten what calm feels like. For burnout and nervous exhaustion. For grief and emotional depletion, when the heart has been asked to bear more than it can hold. For recovery from addiction, particularly supporting the dopamine pathways that addiction dysregulates. For convalescence after illness, when the nervous system needs rebuilding along with everything else. For the "wired but tired" pattern that signals a system that can't turn off because it no longer trusts that rest is safe.

Fresh milky oat tincture is the most potent form for nervous system support. Dried oatstraw - the stalks and leaves - provides excellent minerals but less nervine action. For best results, take milky oat tincture consistently for at least six weeks; twelve weeks is better. This isn't fast medicine. It's rebuilding medicine, and rebuilding takes time.

Milky oats is remarkably safe. It's gluten-free - oats are a different grain than wheat, and the concern about contamination from processing doesn't apply to whole plant preparations. It can be used long-term without concern. It combines beautifully with other nervines, whether you need relaxation or additional tonic support.

Skullcap: The Thought-Quieter

Skullcap is named for the shape of its small, helmet-like flowers, but its medicine is for what happens inside the skull - specifically, for the mind that won't stop. Racing thoughts, circular obsessive thinking, the mental chatter that keeps you awake and exhausted simultaneously - these are skullcap's territory.

Its energetics are cool and bitter, with a deeply relaxing quality. It works quickly enough to provide relief in acute anxiety, yet also builds the nervous system with continued use - an unusual combination that makes it one of the most versatile nervines available. It's both a relaxant you can reach for in moments of crisis and a tonic that strengthens with consistent use.

Skullcap is particularly valuable for anxiety that manifests as mental restlessness - not the physical tension pattern that might call for valerian, but the overactive thinking pattern that won't let you rest. For insomnia driven by a mind that keeps reviewing, planning, worrying, analyzing. For tension headaches that come from mental strain. For those who need calm without heavy sedation, who need to quiet the mind while remaining functional.

Quality matters enormously with skullcap. The herb has been subject to adulteration - substitution with other, cheaper plants that don't have the same properties. Source from reputable suppliers who can verify the identity of their material. Good skullcap works; adulterated product doesn't.

For acute anxiety, skullcap tincture can be taken as needed. For long-term support, consistent daily use over weeks or months builds its tonic effects. It's very safe, without the concerns that accompany stronger sedatives like valerian.

Passionflower: The Gentle Sedative

Passionflower's intricate, otherworldly blossoms seem designed to catch the eye - and perhaps to hint at the plant's capacity to shift consciousness. This is genuine sedative medicine, working on GABA pathways similarly to pharmaceutical anti-anxiety drugs, but with the gentleness that plants offer when pharmaceuticals feel too harsh.

Its energetics are cool and bitter, with a sedating quality that makes it most appropriate for evening use or for acute anxiety that needs genuine calming. Passionflower specifically helps when circular, obsessive thoughts are driving anxiety and preventing sleep. When the mind keeps returning to the same worries, running the same loops, unable to let go and rest - passionflower can break that pattern.

Passionflower is also antispasmodic, helping release nervous tension that has become physical - the tight muscles, the clenched jaw, the gripped belly that chronic anxiety produces. It's been used supportively during withdrawal from sedative medications and sleep drugs, helping ease the transition while the nervous system readjusts.

For anxiety, passionflower tincture can be taken two to three times daily in moderate doses. For sleep, larger doses thirty to sixty minutes before bed help quiet the mind enough for rest to come. As tea, a cup or two before bed provides gentler support.

Because passionflower works on GABA pathways, it may potentiate other sedatives - pharmaceutical or herbal. Avoid driving after taking significant doses. But it's generally very safe, appropriate for regular use during periods of high anxiety or sleep difficulty.

Ashwagandha: The Grounding Adaptogen

Ashwagandha occupies a unique niche among nervine herbs - it's both nervine and adaptogen, both calming and strengthening. Where most adaptogens are stimulating, ashwagandha calms. Where most calming herbs don't build energy, ashwagandha does. This makes it particularly valuable for the modern pattern of exhaustion coexisting with anxiety - the person who is both depleted and unable to rest.

Its energetics are warm, slightly bitter, with a sweet, grounding quality. The root has been used for thousands of years in Ayurvedic medicine, and modern research has validated much of traditional knowledge - ashwagandha genuinely helps the body adapt to stress, supports thyroid function (particularly in hypothyroid patterns), helps restore adrenal function after prolonged stress, and improves sleep quality.

Ashwagandha is specific for the "wired but tired" pattern - exhausted at the core but unable to relax, running on stress hormones because the body doesn't trust that it's safe to stop. It grounds and stabilizes, helping the nervous system shift from sympathetic overdrive toward parasympathetic recovery. Over time, it rebuilds the reserves that chronic stress has depleted.

Traditionally, ashwagandha is taken with warm milk and honey - a preparation sometimes called moon milk - which enhances its grounding, nourishing qualities. It's also available as powder, tincture, or capsules. Consistent use over months produces the best results; this is building medicine, not quick relief.

Ashwagandha belongs to the nightshade family, so those with nightshade sensitivity should be aware, though reactions are rare. It may increase thyroid hormone levels, which is helpful in hypothyroid patterns but potentially problematic for hyperthyroidism. Some caution is warranted with autoimmune conditions, particularly autoimmune thyroid disease. But for most people, ashwagandha is safe for long-term use and profoundly supportive during periods of chronic stress and recovery from burnout.

The Skeletal System: Your Living Foundation

Most people imagine their skeleton as static - a fixed framework that holds them up, unchanging from day to day. But bone is living tissue, constantly being broken down and rebuilt. The skeleton you have today is not the skeleton you had ten years ago; every bone in your body has been remodeled, old tissue removed and new tissue laid down. This continuous reconstruction means that your bones are always responsive to what you provide them - or fail to provide.

Two hundred and six bones make up the adult human skeleton. They provide the structure that keeps you upright, the framework that muscles pull against to create movement. They protect vital organs - skull around brain, ribcage around heart and lungs, pelvis around reproductive organs. They store minerals, particularly calcium and phosphorus, releasing them when the body needs them and rebuilding stores when minerals are plentiful. The marrow within bones produces blood cells - red cells carrying oxygen, white cells defending against infection, platelets enabling clotting.

Bone is roughly two-thirds mineral matrix - calcium phosphate and calcium carbonate crystals providing hardness and rigidity. The other third is organic matrix - primarily collagen, the protein that provides flexibility and resistance to fracture. Without adequate minerals, bones become soft. Without adequate protein, they become brittle. Both components matter.

The constant remodeling of bone is performed by two types of cells working in balance. Osteoclasts break down old bone tissue, creating small cavities. Osteoblasts fill those cavities with new bone material. In healthy bone, these processes balance - what's removed is replaced. When breakdown exceeds building, bone density decreases over time. When building exceeds breakdown, bone density increases. This balance is influenced by hormones, by exercise, by nutrition, by age.

What Bones Need

Healthy bones require a symphony of nutrients working together. Calcium gets the most attention, but it's only one player in a larger ensemble.

Calcium is indeed the primary structural mineral - bones are the body's calcium reservoir. But calcium doesn't work alone. Magnesium works alongside calcium in bone formation and is often deficient in modern diets. Phosphorus combines with calcium to form the mineral crystals that give bone its hardness. Silica strengthens the connective tissue matrix and helps calcium deposit properly. Boron, zinc, and copper support bone formation through various mechanisms. A calcium supplement without these cofactors is addressing only part of the picture.

Vitamins play essential roles. Vitamin D enables calcium absorption - without adequate D, you can consume all the calcium you want and still not get it into your bones. Sunlight on skin triggers vitamin D synthesis, but many people don't get enough sun, particularly in northern latitudes and during winter. Vitamin K2 directs calcium to bones rather than letting it accumulate in arteries - a crucial traffic-directing function found in fermented foods and grass-fed animal products. Vitamin C is essential for collagen synthesis, the protein matrix that gives bone its flexibility.

Protein matters more than most people realize. Bones are one-third protein by weight. Inadequate protein intake means inadequate raw material for the collagen matrix. This is one reason why extreme caloric restriction can damage bone health - the body doesn't have what it needs to rebuild.

Hormones regulate bone metabolism. Estrogen is protective for bone, which is why women's bone density often drops after menopause when estrogen levels fall. Testosterone supports bone density in men. Thyroid and parathyroid hormones regulate calcium metabolism. Chronic cortisol elevation - from prolonged stress or steroid medications - accelerates bone loss.

Weight-bearing exercise is bone's most powerful stimulus. Bones strengthen in response to the mechanical stress of supporting weight and absorbing impact. Walking, hiking, dancing, weight training, yoga - activities where you're bearing weight through your skeleton - signal bones to build density. Swimming and cycling, while excellent for cardiovascular health, don't provide this stimulus because they're not weight-bearing.

Chronic inflammation accelerates bone loss - another reason to address systemic inflammation through diet and lifestyle. Smoking damages bones, as it damages nearly everything. Excessive alcohol interferes with bone formation. Certain medications, particularly corticosteroids and proton pump inhibitors, can compromise bone density with long-term use.

❧ When Bones Weaken

Bone loss happens gradually, silently, without symptoms until it becomes severe. Osteopenia - low bone density - is the precursor stage, a warning that bone loss is outpacing bone building. Osteoporosis is the more advanced condition - bone density so reduced that fractures can occur from minor impacts or even spontaneously. A fall that would merely bruise someone with healthy bones can cause a fracture in someone with osteoporosis.

The consequences of osteoporosis are serious. Hip fractures in the elderly are associated with significant mortality risk - not from the fracture itself, but from the complications that follow immobility. Vertebral compression fractures cause pain and loss of height. Wrist fractures from catching oneself during falls. The fragility that osteoporosis creates limits activity, increases fear, reduces quality of life.

Risk factors include aging, particularly for women after menopause. Poor diet, especially one low in minerals and high in substances that leach them - excessive sugar, phosphoric acid from sodas, too much caffeine. Sedentary lifestyle that doesn't provide the weight-bearing stimulus bones need. Smoking and excessive alcohol. Certain medications used long-term. Family history suggests genetic susceptibility. Small-framed individuals have less bone to lose before reaching dangerous thresholds.

The time to address bone health is before problems develop - building density while the body is still building, maintaining it during middle years, slowing loss as aging makes some loss inevitable. By the time osteoporosis is diagnosed, significant bone mass has already been lost. Prevention is far more effective than treatment.

The Mineral-Rich Herbs

Plants draw minerals from the soil, concentrating them in their tissues. When we prepare these plants appropriately - primarily through long-steeping infusions that have time to extract the minerals - we receive nourishment in a form the body recognizes and can use. This is different from mineral supplements, which provide isolated compounds the body may or may not absorb well. Minerals from plants come with the cofactors and context the body has evolved to work with.

Nettles: The Green Powerhouse

Nettles might be the most mineral-rich plant available to herbalists - a nutritional powerhouse hiding behind a stinging defense. The leaves contain calcium, magnesium, iron, silica, potassium, vitamin K, and a wealth of trace minerals. They also offer protein, chlorophyll, and anti-inflammatory compounds. This isn't a medicinal herb that happens to have nutritional value - it's a food-level source of nutrition with medicinal benefits as well.

Nettles' energetics are cool and dry, with a nutritive, building quality that makes them appropriate for long-term use. They support bone health through their mineral content but also help with anemia (iron), arthritis (anti-inflammatory), allergies (antihistamine effect), and skin health (alterative). They're one of the most broadly useful herbs available, safe enough to drink daily for months or years.

The key to extracting minerals from nettles is time. A quick steep produces a pleasant tea but doesn't pull out the mineral content. A long-steep infusion - four to eight hours, or overnight - extracts what a short steep leaves behind. The resulting liquid is dark, rich, almost broth-like. This is where the medicine is.

To make a nettles infusion: use four to six tablespoons of dried nettles per quart of water. Pour boiling water over the herbs in a quart jar, cover tightly, and let steep for four to eight hours or overnight. Strain and drink two to four cups throughout the day. It can be refrigerated and gently reheated if you prefer it warm. Many people make this a daily practice, preparing a jar each night to drink the next day.

Horsetail: The Silica Source

Horsetail is a primitive plant - a living fossil that has remained essentially unchanged for hundreds of millions of years. Its jointed, segmented stems look nothing like typical herbs, more like something from the age of dinosaurs. What it offers is silica, in quantities no other plant can match.

Silica is essential for connective tissue - the matrix that gives structure to bone, cartilage, skin, hair, and nails. It helps calcium deposit properly in bone rather than in arteries. It supports collagen production. For bone health specifically, silica strengthens the protein matrix that calcium crystals embed in, making bones both strong and flexible rather than just hard and brittle.

Horsetail's energetics are neutral and dry, with an astringent quality that also supports urinary tract health. Beyond bone support, it's used for hair, skin, and nail health - all tissues that depend on silica and collagen for their integrity.

The herb is prepared as decoction or long infusion, one to two cups daily. Unlike nettles, which can be taken indefinitely, horsetail is best used in cycles - six weeks on, two weeks off. Its high silica content can be taxing on the kidneys with continuous long-term use. Those with kidney disease should avoid it. But used cyclically as part of a bone-support program, it provides something no other plant can offer in such concentration.

Oatstraw: Nourishing Both Structure and Nerve

Oatstraw - the dried stalks and leaves of the oat plant, distinct from the milky tops discussed earlier - bridges autumn's two themes beautifully. It provides minerals for bone support and gentle nervine action for nervous system nourishment. This makes it perfect for the season, supporting both foundation and communication simultaneously.

The mineral content includes calcium, magnesium, iron, and silica - a solid contribution to bone health. The nervine action is gentler than the milky tops but still present - calming without sedating, supportive without dramatic effect. Oatstraw's energetics are neutral, sweet, and moist - the qualities of true nourishment.

Oatstraw is prepared as a long-steep infusion, like nettles. It can be combined with nettles, horsetail, and other mineral-rich herbs for a comprehensive bone-support blend. Its mild, slightly sweet flavor makes it pleasant to drink daily over long periods. Very safe for extended use, appropriate for anyone seeking to build mineral reserves and support nervous system health simultaneously.

Red Clover: The Meadow's Gift

Red clover blossoms offer minerals along with something additional - isoflavones, plant compounds that have mild estrogenic activity. This makes red clover particularly relevant for bone health in post-menopausal women, when declining estrogen levels accelerate bone loss. The isoflavones may help partially compensate for this decline, supporting bone density through hormonal as well as nutritional mechanisms.

Beyond bone support, red clover is a classic alterative herb - supporting the body's clearing processes through liver and lymphatic system. Its energetics are cool, moist, and sweet. It's been used traditionally for skin clearing, lymphatic support, and respiratory health.

The flowers are prepared as infusion or tincture. For bone support and general nourishment, two to three cups of infusion daily is appropriate. Red clover combines well with other mineral-rich herbs in bone-support formulas.

The estrogenic activity that makes red clover valuable for post-menopausal bone health is also a reason for caution in hormone-sensitive conditions - estrogen-receptor-positive cancers, endometriosis, fibroids. Those with these conditions should consult with knowledgeable practitioners before using red clover regularly. For most people, it's safe and nourishing.

Beyond Herbs: The Practices That Support Structure

Herbs provide minerals and compounds that support bone health, but they work best alongside practices that give bones the signals they need to build.

Weight-bearing exercise is irreplaceable. Walking is the most accessible - thirty minutes daily provides meaningful stimulus. Hiking, with its uneven terrain and inclines, provides more. Dancing combines weight-bearing with coordination and joy. Weight training directly signals bones to strengthen in response to load. Yoga provides weight-bearing through poses that support body weight against gravity, plus the stretching and balance that reduce fall risk. Choose what you'll actually do; consistency matters more than intensity.

Vitamin D status deserves attention, particularly if you live in northern latitudes or spend most of your time indoors. Have your levels tested; many people are deficient without knowing it. Sunlight on skin is the ideal source, but supplementation may be necessary when sun exposure is limited. Without adequate vitamin D, you can consume all the calcium and minerals you want and still not get them into your bones.

Vitamin K2 directs calcium to bones rather than arteries - an underappreciated role. Fermented foods like natto, sauerkraut, and certain cheeses contain K2. Grass-fed animal products are better sources than conventional ones. Supplements are available for those who don't consume these foods regularly.

Dietary protein provides the raw material for bone's collagen matrix. Adequate protein intake, from whatever sources align with your dietary choices, supports bone rebuilding. Bone broths, if you eat animal products, provide collagen and minerals in a form the body easily uses.

Reducing what leaches minerals makes the minerals you consume go further. Excessive caffeine increases calcium excretion. Sodas, particularly colas with phosphoric acid, disrupt calcium balance. Excessive sugar promotes inflammation that accelerates bone loss. Smoking damages bone along with everything else. Moderating these factors protects the mineral reserves you're working to build.

Embodied Practice: Making a Nourishing Mineral Infusion Blend

This practice invites you to create a mineral-rich herbal blend that you'll use throughout autumn and winter - medicine that nourishes both bones and nervous system, perfect for the season's themes of gathering and grounding. Unlike quick-steeping teas, this blend is designed for long infusion, extracting deep nourishment that short steeps cannot access.

You'll need dried nettles, dried oatstraw, dried horsetail, and optionally dried red clover blossoms. You'll need a container for storing your blend, quart-sized mason jars for making infusions, and a fine strainer. And you'll need the willingness to establish a daily practice of making and drinking your infusion - not as another task on your to-do list, but as a ritual of nourishment.

Read through the entire practice first. Then gather your materials and create your blend with attention and intention.

❧ Meeting the Herbs

Before blending, take time to meet each herb individually. Open your container of nettles and look at the dried leaves - dark green, crumbly, surprisingly light. Smell them - there's a green, slightly earthy quality. If you've ever been stung by fresh nettles, consider how this fierce plant transforms into gentle nourishment when prepared with care.

Open your oatstraw. Notice the pale golden color, the hay-like appearance, the sweet, grassy scent. This is the same plant that feeds horses and becomes oatmeal - humble, nourishing, deeply strengthening.

Look at the horsetail - those strange segmented stems that look like nothing else in the plant kingdom. This ancient plant, virtually unchanged for hundreds of millions of years, offers minerals that no other plant concentrates so powerfully.

If you're including red clover, notice the dried flower heads, still holding hints of pink. These meadow blossoms offer their gentle hormonal support alongside their minerals.

Each of these plants grew from soil, drew minerals up through roots and stems, concentrated what the earth offered into form you can receive. This is what you're preparing to drink.

❧ Blending

A suggested starting ratio: two parts nettles, two parts oatstraw, one part horsetail, one part red clover (if using). But this is a starting point, not a rule. You might adjust based on your particular needs - more oatstraw if nervous system support is your priority, more nettles for iron and broad mineral content, more red clover if you're post-menopausal and seeking additional bone support.

Measure your herbs into a large bowl. Use your hands to blend them together, crumbling any large pieces, mixing until the blend is uniform. As you work, you might consider your intention - what you're building, what reserves you're gathering for the darker months ahead.

Transfer your blend to a glass jar or tin for storage. Label it clearly with contents and date. Stored in a cool, dark place, your blend will remain potent for about a year.

How much to make? A pound of total herbs will last one person about a month of daily use. Make enough for the season, or make smaller batches and replenish as needed.

❧ Making the Daily Infusion

This is the practice you'll return to daily - the ritual of making tomorrow's nourishment today.

In the evening, measure four to six tablespoons of your blend into a quart mason jar. This is more herb than you'd use for regular tea - the long steeping makes this appropriate, extracting minerals that a quick steep would leave behind.

Boil water and pour it over the herbs, filling the jar completely. Cap tightly - this keeps volatile compounds from escaping and allows the infusion to steep without cooling too quickly.

Let the jar sit overnight, or for at least four hours. The long steeping is not optional - it's what makes this medicine rather than just tea. Minerals don't extract quickly; they need time.

In the morning, strain your infusion through a fine strainer. You'll see the color is much darker than quick-steeped tea - deep greenish-brown, almost like a broth. This color tells you the minerals have extracted.

Drink the quart throughout the day - room temperature, gently reheated, or cold from the refrigerator, as you prefer. Some people drink it all in the morning; others sip throughout the day. Find what works for your life.

The spent herbs go to compost. Their minerals have transferred to the water; what remains is fiber with little nutritional value remaining.

❧ The Rhythm of Practice

This daily practice becomes a rhythm - each evening preparing tomorrow's nourishment, each day drinking what you prepared. The rhythm itself is part of the medicine. You're not just consuming minerals; you're building a relationship with nourishment, with preparation, with taking care of yourself in ways that require forethought and intention.

Many people find it helpful to make infusion-preparation part of their evening routine - perhaps while cleaning up after dinner, or as part of winding down for sleep. The act of measuring herbs and pouring hot water can itself become grounding, a moment of presence in the day's transition.

If you miss a day, simply begin again. If you travel and can't maintain the practice, bring the herbs and make infusions where you are, or accept that daily practice isn't always possible and return to it when you're home. The goal is consistency over time, not perfection.

After several weeks of daily use, you may notice changes. Perhaps your energy is more stable. Perhaps your nails are stronger, your hair shinier - signs that minerals are reaching tissues that need them. Perhaps you simply feel more grounded, more resourced, better prepared for winter's demands. The effects are often subtle, accumulating gradually rather than announcing themselves dramatically.

This is autumn's medicine - not dramatic intervention but steady gathering, building reserves that will sustain you through the dark months ahead.

Reflection Questions

1. What is your current nervous system state? Do you recognize the patterns of depletion, overstimulation, chronic sympathetic activation? What does your nervous system actually need?

2. Do you need more relaxation in acute moments, more deep nourishment over time, or both? Which nervine herbs call to you?

3. How is your bone health? Are there risk factors you should be attending to? What practices might support your skeletal foundation?

4. What does it mean to you to "gather" and "ground"? What reserves do you need to build for the darker months ahead?

5. How might you honor autumn's invitation to turn inward, to consolidate, to prepare - even if the culture around you insists on maintaining summer's pace?

6. Where in your life are you in an "autumn" phase - harvesting what you've cultivated, releasing what's complete, preparing for a period of rest or dormancy? How might you work with rather than against this energy?

Autumn teaches: what you gather now sustains you through winter.
Resource your nervous system. Strengthen your bones.
Build your foundation for what lies ahead.

Chapter 8
Winter
Deep Nourishment

The Season of Stillness

Winter is the depth of the cycle - maximum darkness, maximum stillness, the point where everything that rose and bloomed and scattered and gathered finally comes to rest. Seeds lie dormant in frozen ground, looking dead but intensely alive in their waiting. Roots hold stored energy deep in the earth. Bears sleep in their dens, their metabolism slowed to embers. Trees stand bare, their sap descended, their life force concentrated in roots and heartwood. Everything that can rest, rests.

Your body knows this season, even when you ignore it. Energy naturally conserves, wanting to move inward rather than outward. Sleep needs increase with the longer nights - the body asking for more rest in response to more darkness. Appetite often shifts toward warm, dense, nourishing foods - the soups and stews and root vegetables that provide sustained fuel. Metabolism may slow slightly, the body's ancient wisdom knowing that winter was once a time of scarcity requiring conservation. There's a pull toward introspection, dreaming, the inner work that cannot happen while we're busy producing.

But modern humans don't slow. We override seasonal wisdom with artificial light that convinces our bodies it's perpetual summer. We push through fatigue with caffeine and willpower. We maintain the same productivity expectations in December that we had in June. We burn through our deepest reserves - the reserves meant to carry us through scarcity - and then wonder why we're exhausted, depleted, struggling with fertility, aging faster than we should.

Winter asks a radical question: *Can you rest?* Can you do nothing productive and trust that this apparent stillness is itself profoundly productive - the foundation from which all vitality, creativity, and generative capacity arise? Can you stop measuring your worth by your output and allow yourself to lie fallow, to gestate, to dream?

This chapter explores the reproductive system - not just as the mechanics of making babies, but as the deep reservoir of vital energy that underlies all creative capacity. And it explores the medicine of rest itself, which is perhaps winter's most essential teaching.

THE REPRODUCTIVE SYSTEM: THE DEEP RESERVOIR

The reproductive system encompasses far more than reproduction. Yes, it enables conception, pregnancy, and birth. But it also regulates the monthly cycle that organizes so much of female experience. It influences mood, energy, skin, weight, metabolism - threads that weave through daily life regardless of whether you ever intend to conceive. It governs libido and sexual vitality. It shapes the transitions of puberty, perimenopause, and menopause. In men, it maintains testosterone levels across the lifespan, affecting muscle mass, energy, confidence, and sexuality. The reproductive system is the seat of creative life force, whether that force expresses as a child, a work of art, a business, or simply the vitality to meet each day.

This is why reproductive health matters even to those who have no intention of reproducing. The same hormonal balance that enables fertility also enables energy, stable mood, clear skin, healthy weight, and vibrant engagement with life. When reproductive hormones are disrupted, the effects ripple outward into everything.

❧ The Hormonal Dance

Reproductive health depends on a complex interplay of hormones - a dance with many partners, each affecting all the others. Understanding this dance, even in broad strokes, helps you understand why reproductive issues are rarely simple and why addressing them often requires attending to the whole system rather than just one hormone.

The hypothalamus and pituitary gland in the brain form the command center, sending hormonal signals to the ovaries or testes and receiving feedback about what's happening in response. Estrogen, produced primarily by the ovaries, builds the uterine lining each month, maintains bone density, affects mood and cognition, influences skin health. Progesterone, produced after ovulation, maintains pregnancy if conception occurs, balances estrogen's proliferative effects, and has a calming influence on the nervous system. Testosterone, present in all bodies though in different amounts, governs libido, muscle mass, energy, and confidence. FSH and LH, released by the pituitary, regulate ovulation and testosterone production.

But the reproductive hormones don't operate in isolation. Thyroid hormones profoundly affect reproductive function - thyroid disorders commonly disrupt menstrual cycles and fertility. Adrenal hormones, particularly cortisol and DHEA, connect the stress response to reproduction - chronic stress suppresses reproductive function because the body prioritizes survival over reproduction. Insulin, the blood sugar regulating hormone, affects all the other hormones - insulin resistance disrupts the entire hormonal cascade.

What does this intricate system need to function well? Adequate healthy fats, because hormones are literally built from cholesterol. Sufficient calories and nutrients, because the body won't prioritize reproduction if it senses scarcity. Healthy liver function, because the liver metabolizes and clears hormones. Gut health, because gut bacteria participate in estrogen metabolism. Low chronic stress, because the stress axis and reproductive axis are intimately connected. Adequate sleep, because melatonin affects reproductive hormones. Minimal exposure to endocrine-disrupting chemicals, because these synthetic compounds mimic or block hormonal signals.

When any of these factors is significantly off, reproductive health suffers. This is why herbal support for reproductive issues often includes attention to liver, gut, stress response, and nourishment alongside herbs that work directly on reproductive organs.

❧ The Estrobolome: Your Gut's Role in Hormonal Balance

One of the most important and least understood connections in female hormonal health is the relationship between gut bacteria and estrogen. Within the vast community of microbes living in your intestines, a specific subset - collectively called the estrobolome - directly participates in estrogen metabolism. These bacteria produce an enzyme called beta-glucuronidase that influences how much estrogen your body retains versus how much it eliminates. This makes gut health not just generally important, but specifically crucial for estrogen balance.

Here's how it works: when the liver processes estrogen for elimination, it attaches a molecule to the estrogen through a process called conjugation, essentially tagging it for removal. This conjugated estrogen travels via bile into the intestines, destined to leave the body through the stool. But beta-glucuronidase, produced by certain gut bacteria, can remove that tag - unconjugating the estrogen and allowing it to be reabsorbed back into circulation rather than eliminated.

When the estrobolome is balanced, an appropriate amount of estrogen recirculates and an appropriate amount leaves. But when gut bacteria are imbalanced - a state called dysbiosis - beta-glucuronidase activity may be too high, causing excessive estrogen to recirculate. This contributes to estrogen dominance, a pattern underlying many common hormonal issues: heavy and painful periods, PMS, fibrocystic breasts, fibroids, endometriosis, and increased risk of estrogen-sensitive cancers.

Conversely, when the microbiome lacks diversity or when beneficial bacteria are depleted, beta-glucuronidase may be too low, allowing too much estrogen to leave. This can contribute to symptoms of low estrogen - vaginal dryness, bone loss, mood changes - even when the ovaries are producing adequate amounts.

What disrupts the estrobolome? Many of the same things that disrupt the microbiome generally: antibiotic use, chronic stress, poor diet (particularly low fiber and high sugar), environmental toxins, and chronic inflammation. What supports it? A diverse, fiber-rich diet that feeds beneficial bacteria. Fermented foods that introduce helpful microbes. Adequate prebiotic foods - garlic, onions, leeks, asparagus, Jerusalem artichokes - that nourish the microbes already present. Reducing unnecessary antibiotic exposure. Managing stress, which directly affects gut bacteria composition.

This is why digestive health is so often relevant to hormonal issues that seem unrelated to digestion. A woman struggling with estrogen dominance - heavy periods, breast tenderness, fibroids - may need to address her gut as much as her reproductive organs. The bitter herbs that support liver function also support healthy bile flow, which matters for estrogen elimination. The fiber in a whole-foods diet doesn't just support bowel regularity; it feeds the bacteria that regulate estrogen. The stress management that calms the nervous system also helps maintain the gut environment where hormonal balance is negotiated.

The body is not a collection of separate systems; it's a web of relationships. Hormonal health depends on gut health. Gut health depends on what you eat, how you manage stress, and whether you've maintained microbial diversity. Everything connects.

❧ The Monthly Cycle

A healthy menstrual cycle is regular - twenty-one to thirty-five days, consistent for that particular person even if different from average. It's not excessively painful; mild cramping is normal, but debilitating pain that interferes with daily life is not. Bleeding is moderate - three to seven days, not flooding through protection or barely present. Premenstrual changes are minimal; some body awareness is normal, but severe mood swings, breast tenderness, bloating, and irritability indicate imbalance. For those tracking fertility signs, cervical mucus changes and temperature shifts are clear and predictable.

When cycles don't fit this picture, something is asking for attention. PMS - that collection of mood changes, physical discomfort, and general misery in the days before bleeding - often reflects progesterone insufficiency, liver congestion, or chronic stress. Painful periods may indicate excess inflammation, uterine tension, or conditions like endometriosis that require medical evaluation. Heavy bleeding can result from hormonal imbalance or from structural issues like fibroids or polyps that need to be ruled out. Irregular cycles - unpredictable timing, sometimes long, sometimes short - often reflect stress, thyroid issues, or conditions like polycystic ovarian syndrome. Absent periods can result from extreme stress, very low body fat, hormonal disorders, or simply being out of balance in ways that make the body unwilling to ovulate.

Herbal support for menstrual health focuses on several strategies: supporting hormonal balance, often by encouraging adequate progesterone production or helping the body modulate estrogen levels; reducing inflammation and cramping; supporting liver clearance of excess hormones; nourishing and toning the reproductive organs; and addressing stress, which underlies so many hormonal issues. The herbs that follow work through various combinations of these strategies.

Meeting the Reproductive Herbs

Raspberry Leaf: The Uterine Toner

Raspberry leaf is the great uterine tonic of Western herbalism - gentle, nourishing, safe enough for daily use throughout life. The leaves of the common raspberry plant, dried and infused, provide medicine that strengthens and tones the muscular tissue of the uterus without stimulating contractions. This toning action makes the uterus work more efficiently at whatever it's doing - contracting during menstruation, contracting during labor, recovering after birth.

Its energetics are neutral, slightly dry, with an astringent quality that tightens and tones tissue. Beyond its uterine affinity, raspberry leaf is mineral-rich - iron, calcium, magnesium - providing nutritive support alongside its toning action.

For menstrual cramping, raspberry leaf works not by suppressing the cramping reflex but by improving the coordination of uterine muscle contractions. A toned muscle contracts more efficiently and with less pain than a flaccid one. For heavy bleeding, its astringent quality helps reduce excessive flow. For pregnancy, traditional use throughout the second and third trimesters prepares the uterus for the demanding work of labor. For postpartum recovery, it supports the uterus in returning to its pre-pregnancy state.

Raspberry leaf is typically taken as infusion - two to four cups daily throughout the cycle for menstrual support, or throughout the later stages of pregnancy for birth preparation. It's very safe, gentle enough for daily long-term use. The traditional caution about avoiding it in the first trimester of pregnancy is not based on evidence of harm but on general caution during the vulnerable early weeks; most practitioners consider it safe throughout pregnancy, though some prefer to wait until the second trimester.

Vitex: The Cycle Regulator

Vitex, also called chaste tree berry, works differently from most reproductive herbs - rather than acting directly on the reproductive organs, it acts on the pituitary gland in the brain, influencing the hormonal signals that regulate the entire cycle. This makes it one of the most powerful herbs for addressing hormonal imbalance, but also one that requires patience and commitment to see results.

Its energetics are slightly warm and drying, with a pungent quality. The berries contain compounds that influence pituitary function, particularly increasing the release of luteinizing hormone (LH), which in turn supports progesterone production after ovulation. Vitex also lowers prolactin levels, which can be helpful for certain types of breast tenderness and some fertility challenges.

Vitex is specific for patterns involving insufficient progesterone - the short luteal phase, the PMS that hits hard in the second half of the cycle, the irregular cycles that suggest ovulation isn't happening reliably. For these patterns, vitex can be remarkably effective. But it's not a universal solution for all menstrual issues; it works best for specific hormonal patterns and may not help (or may even aggravate) patterns with different underlying causes.

The key to using vitex is consistency and patience. It must be taken daily, ideally first thing in the morning, for at least three to six months to see its full effects. The pituitary is slow to shift; you're essentially retraining the hormonal command center, and that takes time. Starting vitex and stopping after a few weeks because you don't see results misses how this herb works.

Vitex should not be used during pregnancy - it's for regulating cycles and supporting conception, not for use once conception has occurred. It may interact with hormonal birth control. It affects dopamine pathways, so caution is warranted with certain psychiatric medications. And it's not appropriate for everyone; some people respond well, others don't, and a small number feel worse. If vitex doesn't seem to be helping after several months of consistent use, it may not be the right herb for your particular pattern.

Cramp Bark: The Muscle Relaxer

Cramp bark does exactly what its name suggests - it relaxes cramping muscles. This includes the smooth muscle of the uterus, making it one of the most reliably effective herbs for menstrual cramps. It also relaxes skeletal muscle, helping with the back spasms, leg cramps, and general muscle tension that often accompany painful periods.

Its energetics are neutral and bitter, with both antispasmodic and mild nervine qualities. The bark of this shrub - a viburnum relative of the ornamental snowball bush - contains compounds that directly relax muscle tissue. Unlike pain medications that mask the sensation of cramping while the muscles continue to spasm, cramp bark addresses the spasm itself.

For acute menstrual cramping, cramp bark tincture can be taken at the first sign of discomfort - and this is key, because catching cramps early prevents the cascade of tension and pain that becomes harder to interrupt once established. The dose can be repeated every fifteen to thirty minutes until relief is achieved, then continued at longer intervals as needed. For those with predictably painful periods, starting cramp bark a day before bleeding typically begins can prevent cramps from developing their full intensity.

Cramp bark is also used for threatened miscarriage when uterine spasms are causing concern - though this application belongs in the hands of experienced practitioners working alongside medical care, not in self-treatment.

The herb is very safe, with the only significant caution being for those with aspirin sensitivity, as cramp bark contains salicylates. Tincture is the most common and effective preparation for acute cramping; the taste is bitter but tolerable, and the relief is usually worth it.

Dong Quai: The Blood Nourisher

Dong quai holds a revered place in East Asian medicine as the primary blood tonic for women - sometimes called "female ginseng" for its nourishing, building qualities. Its approach to reproductive health is fundamentally different from herbs like vitex; rather than modulating hormones directly, dong quai nourishes and builds the blood, improves circulation to the reproductive organs, and supports the body's own capacity for balance.

Its energetics are warm, sweet, and moistening - the qualities of building and nourishing. The root has an affinity for blood, helping address the depletion that comes from menstruation itself, supporting recovery from blood loss, and nourishing the tissues that depend on good blood supply.

Dong quai is traditionally used for patterns involving blood deficiency - scanty periods, pale complexion, fatigue that worsens with menstruation, recovery from childbirth or blood loss. It eases cramping by improving circulation to the uterus, relaxing tissue that's tense from inadequate blood supply. For menopause, particularly when dryness is a prominent symptom, dong quai's moistening quality provides relief.

In traditional practice, dong quai is rarely used alone; it's typically combined with other herbs in formulas tailored to specific patterns. When used for menstrual support, it's often taken during the follicular phase - after bleeding ends until ovulation - the building phase of the cycle when its nourishing qualities are most appropriate.

Dong quai should not be used during pregnancy, as it can stimulate uterine contractions. It should not be used during heavy menstrual bleeding, as it may increase flow. Those on blood-thinning medications should use caution, as dong quai contains coumarins that may compound anticoagulant effects. It may increase sensitivity to sunlight in some people. These are real cautions, but for the right patterns and situations, dong quai offers profound nourishment.

MENOPAUSE: THE WISDOM TRANSITION

Menopause is not a disease to be treated but a profound life transition to be supported. The end of reproductive years marks the beginning of something else - what many traditions call the wisdom years, when the energy once devoted to reproduction becomes available for other forms of creativity, leadership, and service. The crone, the wise woman, the elder who has passed through the gate - these archetypes honor what begins when fertility ends.

But the transition itself - perimenopause, the years surrounding the final period - can be genuinely challenging. Hormones fluctuate unpredictably as the ovaries wind down their decades of cyclic production. Hot flashes and night sweats disrupt sleep and daily life. Vaginal tissue thins and dries, making intercourse uncomfortable. Sleep becomes elusive just when it's most needed. Mood shifts - irritability, anxiety, depression - arrive without obvious cause. Cognition may feel foggy, memory less reliable. Bone density begins declining as estrogen's protective effect withdraws. Cardiovascular risk increases. Weight redistributes in frustrating ways.

These symptoms are not inevitable - some women sail through menopause with minimal disruption - but they're common enough that most women experience at least some of them. They're not signs of weakness or failure; they're signs of a body navigating a significant hormonal shift.

Herbal support for menopause includes herbs that address specific symptoms and herbs that support the body's overall adaptation. Black cohosh is the best-studied herb for hot flashes, helping many women reduce their frequency and intensity. Sage, that common kitchen herb, has traditional use for reducing excessive sweating and hot flashes. Motherwort calms heart palpitations and eases the anxiety that often accompanies perimenopause. Red clover offers mild phytoestrogens along with mineral support for bones. Vitex can be helpful in early perimenopause when cycles are still present but irregular. Shatavari, cooling and moistening, addresses the dryness that affects vaginal tissue, skin, and often the whole system. Adaptogens like ashwagandha and holy basil support the stress response, which is often heightened during this transition.

Beyond herbs specifically for menopausal symptoms, this transition calls for the support explored in earlier chapters - mineral-rich herbs for bones, hawthorn and cardiovascular support, nervines for the nervous system that's being asked to adapt to a new hormonal reality. Menopause is not a single issue to address but a whole-body transition that benefits from comprehensive support.

The invitation of menopause is to step into the wise woman years with intention - to grieve what is ending, to honor what was, and to welcome what becomes possible when reproductive energy transforms into something new.

Adaptogens for Deep Reserves

Winter is the season for adaptogens - those remarkable herbs that help the body adapt to stress while building deep reserves of vitality. Unlike stimulants that push the body to perform beyond its resources, adaptogens work by increasing the body's capacity to handle challenge without depleting its foundations. They're building herbs, nourishing herbs, the kind of medicine that works slowly over months to create lasting resilience.

Shatavari: The Nurturer

Shatavari - whose name translates evocatively as "she who has a hundred husbands" - is the primary reproductive tonic for women in Ayurvedic medicine. Where ashwagandha is warming and grounding, shatavari is cooling and moistening, making it particularly valuable for those who run hot and dry, and for the menopausal transition when dryness often predominates.

Its energetics are cool, sweet, and deeply nourishing. The root supports fertility, eases menopausal symptoms, promotes lactation in nursing mothers, and generally nurtures the female reproductive system through all its phases. But its gifts extend beyond reproduction - shatavari moistens dry tissues throughout the body, soothes irritated digestive tracts, and cools inflammatory conditions.

As an adaptogen, shatavari helps the body adapt to stress while building rather than depleting reserves. It's gentle enough for long-term daily use, working gradually over weeks and months to restore what chronic stress has consumed. For those who feel burned out, dried out, running on empty - shatavari offers slow, steady replenishment.

The root is taken as powder (traditionally mixed with warm milk and honey), as tincture, or in capsules. Consistent daily use over extended periods produces the best results.

Reishi: The Spirit Nourisher

Reishi mushroom has been revered for millennia in East Asian traditions as the "mushroom of immortality" - not because it literally grants eternal life, but because it nourishes the spirit and builds the kind of deep vitality that supports a long, healthy life. In the winter season, when darkness invites us inward and the spirit needs tending, reishi offers its gentle, profound support.

Reishi calms the mind and supports deep, restorative sleep - not through sedation but through nourishing the nervous system and helping it find its natural rhythm. It modulates immune function, neither stimulating nor suppressing but helping the immune system self-regulate. It protects the liver, that organ of transformation that works so hard to process everything we encounter. And it nourishes what's sometimes called shen - spirit, consciousness, the quality of presence and peace that allows us to meet life with equanimity.

For those going through difficult times - grief, major transitions, periods of uncertainty - reishi offers support that goes beyond the physical. It's medicine for the spirit as much as for the body, helping us find ground when everything feels unstable.

Reishi is taken as decoction (the dried mushroom simmered for hours), as extract, or as powder added to drinks. It's very safe, gentle enough for daily use over years. Its flavor is bitter and earthy - not unpleasant to those who appreciate it, but not everyone's favorite. Adding it to coffee, cacao, or blending with other herbs can make it more palatable.

Holy Basil: The Uplifting Adaptogen

Holy basil - tulsi in Sanskrit - is held sacred in Ayurvedic tradition, planted at household shrines and honored daily. Its medicine is uplifting and clarifying, supporting stress resilience while maintaining mental clarity and even elevating mood. Where some adaptogens are grounding and sedating, holy basil is enlivening without being stimulating - a rare and valuable quality.

Holy basil supports the body's stress response, helping maintain balance when demands are high. It has beneficial effects on blood sugar regulation, making it supportive for the metabolic disruption that chronic stress often causes. It supports respiratory health and has antimicrobial properties. And it simply tastes good - fragrant, slightly spicy, pleasant as a daily tea in a way that makes consistent use easy.

As a daily tea - two or three cups throughout the day - holy basil provides gentle adaptogenic support that accumulates over time. It can also be taken as tincture. It combines beautifully with other adaptogens, adding its uplifting quality to formulas that might otherwise be too heavy or sedating.

The Medicine of Rest

Modern culture worships productivity. We wear exhaustion as a badge of honor, humble-bragging about how busy we are, how little we slept, how much we accomplished despite running on empty. Rest is seen as laziness, weakness, the refuge of those who can't keep up. We'll rest when we're dead, we say, not recognizing that we're hastening that arrival by refusing to rest while we're alive.

But rest is not the absence of productivity. Rest is when the real work happens. During sleep, muscles repair and grow stronger. The immune system strengthens, producing the cells and antibodies that protect you. Hormones balance, doing their regulatory work free from the interference of daytime stress. Memories consolidate and learning integrates, the brain processing what was encountered during waking hours. Creativity emerges from the unconscious, problems solving themselves while you dream. The nervous system resets from the day's stress, restoring the capacity to handle tomorrow's challenges. Cellular repair and waste clearance occur, maintaining the tissues that keep you functioning. The spirit is nourished, replenished, made whole.

Without adequate rest, all of this suffers. Chronic fatigue becomes the baseline. Hormones drift out of balance, affecting mood, weight, fertility, and resilience. Immunity weakens, and every cold that passes through finds a home in your depleted body. Mental health deteriorates - anxiety and depression feed on exhaustion. Burnout arrives, the body finally refusing to continue what the will insisted upon.

Aging accelerates, the repair processes falling behind the damage. Deep reserves deplete, the vitality that should carry you through decades consumed in years.

Winter teaches what we refuse to learn the rest of the year: productivity comes *from* rest, not despite it. The seed cannot grow if it never stops moving. The field cannot produce if it's never left fallow. The body cannot thrive if it's never allowed to restore. Rest is not the opposite of productivity; rest is the foundation of productivity. Everything that rises must first gather itself in stillness.

❧ Honoring Winter in a Culture That Won't Stop

Most of us cannot fully honor winter's invitation to rest. We have jobs that demand the same output in December as in June. We have responsibilities that don't pause for the season. We live in heated, lit environments that insulate us from the natural cues that would slow us down. Complete hibernation isn't possible.

But partial honor is still honor. Small shifts toward winter's rhythm, accumulated over the dark months, still make a difference. Going to bed earlier - even thirty minutes earlier - when the body is asking for more sleep. Saying no to some of the social obligations that pack the holiday season. Choosing the warm bath over the extra hour of work. Eating the nourishing soup instead of grabbing something fast. Taking the walk in daylight when daylight is scarce, feeding the body's need for natural light and gentle movement.

Winter's nourishment includes the warm, dense, cooked foods that provide sustained fuel - soups and stews, root vegetables, healthy fats that the body craves when warmth is scarce. It includes adequate protein, because building and repair require raw materials. It includes the mineral-rich infusions from autumn, continued through winter to maintain the reserves you built.

And winter's nourishment includes the adaptogens - taken consistently through the dark months, rebuilding deep reserves, supporting the body's capacity to handle whatever stress remains even as you try to reduce it. This is the season for reishi in your evening drink, for ashwagandha or shatavari in your morning routine, for holy basil tea in the afternoon. Not as stimulation, not as performance enhancement, but as deep feeding of a body that has given much and needs replenishment.

When to Seek Medical Care

Herbs support reproductive health beautifully, but they work best alongside appropriate medical care, not instead of it. Know when the situation calls for professional evaluation.

Severe or worsening menstrual issues - pain that's getting worse over time, bleeding that's become unmanageable, symptoms that don't respond to reasonable interventions - may indicate conditions like fibroids, endometriosis, or polycystic ovarian syndrome that need diagnosis and often benefit from medical treatment. Sudden changes in an established cycle - particularly mid-cycle bleeding, bleeding after menopause, or a period that simply stops - warrant evaluation to rule out concerning causes. Very heavy bleeding with large clots, or any bleeding that's causing symptoms of anemia, needs attention.

Fertility challenges benefit from medical assessment alongside herbal support - understanding what's happening physiologically guides more effective intervention. Suspected pregnancy should be confirmed and prenatal care established. Abnormal bleeding patterns - between periods, after intercourse, or after menopause - require evaluation.

Serious chronic fatigue that doesn't improve with rest and reasonable self-care may indicate thyroid dysfunction, autoimmune conditions, anemia, or other issues that need diagnosis and appropriate treatment.

Herbal medicine and medical care are not opponents. They work beautifully together, each offering what the other cannot. Know when to reach for herbs, and know when to seek additional help.

Chapter 9

Celestial Rhythms and the Art of Timing

Wheels Within Wheels

We have moved through the wheel of the year - spring's rising, summer's fullness, autumn's gathering, winter's depth. These seasonal rhythms organize our relationship with plants and with our own bodies across the span of months. But within the year, smaller wheels turn. The moon completes her cycle roughly thirteen times while the earth circles the sun once. Each lunar month contains its own arc of beginning, building, culmination, and release - a complete journey from darkness through light and back to darkness, happening again and again within the larger journey of the seasons.

The alchemists knew this. They called the moon *Luna*, associated her with silver, with water, with the feminine principle, with the realm of dreams and intuition. They understood that solar and lunar were two modes of knowing - the sun illuminating what can be seen directly, the moon revealing what can only be glimpsed by reflection. To work with plants was to work with both: the solar force of photosynthesis that builds plant bodies from light, and the lunar force that draws water upward through stems, that times flowering and fruiting, that pulls at the sap the way she pulls at the sea.

Modern life has largely severed our awareness of these rhythms. Electric light makes the moon's phases irrelevant to our activities. We can read, work, travel regardless of whether she shines or hides. Climate-controlled environments insulate us from the seasonal shifts she once amplified. Clocks and schedules override the body's natural responses to her presence or absence. We can live as if time were uniform, every hour like every other, every night interchangeable.

But the rhythms continue whether we attend to them or not. The moon still pulls the tides. Sap still rises and falls in response to her call. Hormones still cycle in patterns older than our species. Seeds still know, somehow, what phase she wears. We can ignore these rhythms, but we cannot escape them. We are *of* this earth, and this earth dances with the moon.

When we choose to align with lunar rhythms rather than override them, something shifts - not just in effectiveness, but in our experience of being alive in a living cosmos. We remember that we are not separate from nature, managing it from outside, but participants in something vast and ancient that includes us whether we acknowledge it or not. This remembering is itself a kind of medicine.

The Closest Celestial Presence

Of all the celestial bodies, the moon is nearest to us - close enough that her gravitational pull visibly moves the waters of our planet twice each day. Stand at the ocean's edge and watch the tide come in; you are watching the moon's embrace of the earth made visible. This is not metaphor. The physics are real. But physics does not exhaust what the moon is or what she offers.

She is also presence. Walk outside on a full moon night and feel her light on your skin, silver and cool, different in quality from sunlight in ways that go beyond wavelength and intensity. Something in you responds - something old, something that knew the moon before it knew language. Poets have tried to capture this for millennia; none have fully succeeded. The moon speaks to a part of us that predates words.

The tides demonstrate her physical influence beyond any doubt. The question is not whether the moon affects the ocean - that is simply observed fact - but how far her influence extends. Does she also pull at the water in soil, drawing moisture upward through earth? Does she call to the sap in trees, timing its rise and fall? Does she whisper to the fluids in animal bodies, in human bodies - the blood, the lymph, the cerebrospinal fluid that bathes the brain?

Traditional peoples around the world answered yes. Not from theory but from observation, accumulated over generations, encoded into practice because it worked. They noticed that plants harvested at certain moon phases kept better, dried more easily, seemed to hold more potency. They observed that wounds bled more at some times than others, that healing seemed to follow lunar rhythms. They tracked fertility and birth and death against the moon's phases and found correlations too consistent to ignore.

Modern science has investigated some of these observations, confirmed a few, failed to confirm others, and largely ignored most. The mechanistic framework that dominates research has little room for influences that can't be isolated into single variables and measured in controlled conditions. But absence of scientific proof is not proof of absence. And the kind of knowing that comes from generations of direct observation, from bodies attuned to rhythms through necessity rather than choice, is its own form of evidence - perhaps less precise than laboratory data, but in some ways deeper.

You are invited into relationship with the moon - not as belief system requiring your faith, but as living presence you can come to know through attention. Watch her. Track her. Notice what shifts in you and around you as she waxes and wanes. The moon has been offering this teaching since before there were humans to receive it. She asks nothing but your willingness to look up.

The Tidal Body

Your body is mostly water. Not metaphorically - literally. Roughly sixty percent of your weight is water. Your brain floats in fluid, is composed of fluid. Your blood is water carrying everything the body needs to move from place to place. Your cells are tiny seas, their membranes the shores. You are, in the most physical sense, a body of water shaped like a person.

And water responds to the moon. Not only ocean water - all water. The forces are subtler in smaller bodies, in contained bodies, but they don't disappear. The moon pulls at the water in lakes, in rivers, in the glass on your nightstand - and in you. Microtides move through every fluid in your body, too subtle to feel directly but present nonetheless, part of the constant flux that is being alive.

What might these microtides mean for physiology? Traditional medicine systems were certain they mattered. Ayurvedic practitioners considered the moon's phases when prescribing treatments, believing the body's receptivity to medicine shifted across the lunar month. European folk healers avoided surgery at certain moon phases, having observed that bleeding was harder to control. Women in countless cultures tracked their bleeding against the moon, finding rhythms that gave meaning and predictability to their cycles.

Modern research, when it bothers to look, finds hints that these traditions weren't imaginary. Studies have found correlations between lunar phases and sleep quality - people sleeping less and less deeply around full moon, even in controlled environments without moonlight exposure, as if the body knows the moon's phase without seeing it. Research suggests variations in cardiovascular function, in hormone levels, in the timing of births. The evidence is inconsistent - some studies find effects, others don't - but the pattern of findings suggests something is happening, even if we don't fully understand what or why.

Perhaps more interesting than any study is what happens when you begin tracking your own experience against the moon's phases. Keep notes for several months and see what patterns emerge. Many people discover correlations they hadn't noticed - sleep shifting, energy rising and falling, moods patterning in lunar rhythm. This isn't proof of anything, but it's *your* experience, and your experience matters.

The most profound correlation may be the menstrual cycle - roughly 29.5 days matching the moon's synodic month, the very word "menstruation" from the Latin for moon. Studies of women living without artificial light show stronger synchronization between cycles and lunar phases, suggesting the correlation may be more than coincidence - that the human cycle evolved in relationship with the moon and that electric light has disrupted what was once a natural attunement. Some women who begin tracking both cycles find them drifting into alignment over time, as if the body remembers a relationship it had forgotten.

You are a tidal being, whether you feel it or not. Your waters rise and fall with rhythms older than humanity. The invitation is simply to begin feeling it - to pay attention, over months and cycles, to how you move through the lunar month. Your own observation is valid. Your own experience is data.

The Lunar Cycle: A Journey Through Light and Shadow

The moon's cycle from new to full and back to new spans approximately 29.5 days - one complete journey from darkness through maximum light and back to darkness. This is an alchemical arc, a story of emergence and return, of manifestation and dissolution. Understanding this arc as more than astronomy - as living rhythm with its own intelligence - helps you work with energies that are already in motion rather than pushing against the current.

☽○☾ The Dark Moon and New Moon: The Seed in the Dark

The new moon is invisible. She hangs between earth and sun, her illuminated face turned away from us, offering nothing but darkness to the night sky. This is the void point, the pause between breaths, the moment of maximum potential before anything emerges. In alchemical terms, this is the *nigredo* - the blackening, the necessary darkness from which all transformation begins.

The dark moon days - the two or three days surrounding the new moon - carry this energy of withdrawal, of incubation, of seeds gestating beneath frozen soil. Life force is concentrated inward and downward. In plants, sap is at its lowest point in stems and leaves, pooled in roots. In bodies, energy may feel contracted, dreamy, less available for external demands. This is not emptiness to be filled but fullness of a different kind - the fullness of potential not yet expressed.

What wants to begin at new moon? What seeds are you planting, literally or metaphorically? This is the time for intention-setting, for initiating what you want to grow. It's also a time for rest, for retreat, for honoring the part of you that needs darkness the way seeds need darkness - not as absence but as necessary condition for what comes next.

For herbal work, new moon favors planting, especially root crops that will grow downward into the earth. It favors beginning inward practices - starting a journal, committing to a meditation practice, initiating internal work. It's generally not considered ideal for harvesting aerial parts of plants, as the vital force is drawn down into roots rather than expressed in leaves and flowers. But it may be a powerful time for harvesting roots themselves, or for beginning preparations meant to support deep, inward processes.

☽○☾ The Waxing Moon: Rising Into Light

As the first sliver of light appears and grows night by night, we enter the waxing phase - the moon's journey from darkness toward fullness. Each evening she shows more of her face, stays longer in the sky, grows in power and presence. Something is building. The darkness has yielded its gift, and now that gift rises into visibility.

Waxing moon energy is expansive, outward-moving, gathering momentum. In plants, sap rises. Water moves upward through stems. Life force concentrates in the parts above ground - leaves reaching, buds forming, flowers preparing to open. In bodies, energy often increases. What was planted at new moon begins to grow; projects gain traction; what you're calling toward you comes closer.

This is the phase for building, for increase, for feeding what you want to grow. Work that requires energy and initiative is supported. Courage may come more easily. The world feels more receptive to effort, more willing to meet you halfway.

For herbal work, waxing moon favors planting crops that fruit above ground. It's considered optimal for harvesting leaves, flowers, and aerial parts, as sap is rising and vital force is moving upward into exactly those parts. Tinctures and preparations meant to build, strengthen, or increase are well-begun during this phase, their extraction process mirroring the moon's own building toward fullness.

☽○☾ The Full Moon: The Illuminated Peak

The full moon stands opposite the sun, her entire face bathed in reflected light, bright enough to read by, powerful enough to stir the blood. This is the culmination - everything that was building has built; everything that was rising has risen. The tide is highest. The sap has peaked. Whatever was hidden in darkness now stands fully illuminated.

Full moon energy is intense, externalized, sometimes overwhelming. Emergency rooms staff up; teachers report more chaotic classrooms; sensitive people may feel the surge as restlessness, insomnia, heightened emotion. This is maximum expression - and maximum expression can tip into excess. The very fullness can feel like too much.

But fullness is also celebration, revelation, the joy of culmination. What you've been building reaches its peak. What was obscure becomes clear. Full moon illuminates - sometimes uncomfortably, showing what we'd rather not see, but illuminating nonetheless. There's a reason rituals of release and revelation cluster around the full moon; she shows everything, hiding nothing.

In plants, water content peaks. Sap is at its highest in stems and leaves. This makes full moon less ideal for harvesting herbs meant for drying - the extra moisture means more effort to dry completely and more risk of mold. But for fresh plant preparations - juices, fresh tinctures, poultices - full moon harvest captures maximum vitality. The plant is most fully itself, most fully expressed.

For your own practice, full moon invites acknowledgment of what has been accomplished, celebration of what has reached fullness, and sometimes release of what the illumination reveals as no longer needed. Stand in her light if you can. Let yourself be seen by the moon.

☽○☾ The Waning Moon: The Return to Darkness

From fullness, the moon begins her descent - each night a little less light, a little more shadow eating into the bright disk. The waning phase is the journey back toward darkness, the other half of the cycle, the exhale after the inhale. What rose now falls. What expanded now contracts. The tide recedes.

Waning moon energy is contracting, inward-moving, releasing. In plants, sap descends. Life force withdraws from above-ground parts back into roots and seeds. In bodies, energy may turn inward. There's a natural pull toward completion, toward finishing what was started, toward letting go of what has served its purpose.

This is the phase for decrease - for breaking habits, clearing clutter, releasing relationships or patterns that no longer serve. What you want less of, attend to during the waning moon. Cleansing practices, physical and spiritual, are supported. The energy is moving toward the void point of new moon; use it to empty what needs emptying.

For herbal work, waning moon is the traditional time for root harvest. The vital force has descended; the root holds the plant's concentrated essence. It's a good time for pruning and weeding -

removing what you don't want while the energy favors decrease. Preparations meant to release, cleanse, or clear are well-begun now, their purpose aligned with the moon's own movement toward emptiness.

As the moon thins toward invisible, we approach the dark moon again - the completion of the cycle, the return to the seed point, the pause before the next beginning. Honor this ending. Rest in the darkness. Trust that what needs to emerge will emerge when the time is right.

Plants and the Moon

Plants are rooted. They cannot move toward what they need or away from what threatens them. This fixed nature has made them exquisitely sensitive to the rhythms that flow through them - light and darkness, warmth and cold, moisture and drought, the pull of gravity, and perhaps the pull of the moon.

Traditional agricultural knowledge around the world incorporates lunar timing with a consistency that suggests these practices emerged independently, from direct observation, across cultures that had no contact with each other. Plant root crops when the moon is waning and sap descending. Plant leafy crops when the moon is waxing and sap rising. Harvest what grows above ground when lunar force is pulling upward; harvest what grows below ground when it's pulling downward. The specifics vary, but the basic recognition - that the moon matters for planting and harvesting - is remarkably universal.

What do the plants themselves experience? We can't know directly - plants don't report their inner states - but we can observe their behavior. Some research has found correlations between lunar phase and germination rates. Some studies have tracked variations in leaf movement, in growth rate, in the timing of water uptake. The results are suggestive rather than conclusive, but they align with what traditional farmers have always claimed: the moon's phase matters for plant growth.

Perhaps more important than research findings is what you can observe yourself. Plant the same seeds at different moon phases and watch what happens. Harvest the same herb at full moon and at waning moon, dry them separately, taste them, work with them, notice if you perceive any difference. Your garden and your medicine-making are not laboratories in the scientific sense, but they are laboratories for your own knowing - places where you can develop direct relationship with these rhythms rather than taking anyone's word for what they mean.

The traditional guidelines for lunar harvesting make intuitive sense if we accept that sap rises and falls with the moon. For leaves, flowers, and aerial parts, harvest during waxing moon when sap is rising, or near full moon when it has risen. The plant's energy is concentrated in exactly the parts you're harvesting. Morning is generally preferred - after dew has dried but before afternoon heat volatilizes the aromatics. The plant is awake, turgid, expressing itself fully in its above-ground parts.

For roots, harvest during waning moon when sap has descended, when the plant has withdrawn its energy into its underground parts. Autumn harvest aligns both lunar and seasonal rhythms - the plant dying back above ground, concentrating its essence below, the moon pulling downward as you dig. The root you harvest holds what the plant has been gathering all season.

These are guidelines, not commandments. A plant harvested at the "wrong" moon phase is still medicine. What matters most is harvesting with attention, with gratitude, with awareness of the plant as living being offering part of itself for your use. But when you can align your harvesting with lunar rhythms, you add another layer of relationship - not just with the plant, but with the celestial influence that has been shaping plant life since long before humans existed to notice.

BIODYNAMIC PRACTICE: READING THE CELESTIAL GARDEN

Biodynamic agriculture, developed by Rudolf Steiner in the 1920s, offers one systematic framework for working with cosmic influences on plants. It extends lunar awareness to include planetary positions and zodiacal signs, creating an intricate calendar for planting, cultivating, and harvesting that reads the heavens for guidance on earthly work.

In the biodynamic system, the zodiac divides into four elemental groups: earth signs (Taurus, Virgo, Capricorn), water signs (Cancer, Scorpio, Pisces), air signs (Gemini, Libra, Aquarius), and fire signs (Aries, Leo, Sagittarius). As the moon moves through each sign - spending roughly two and a half days in each - different aspects of plant growth are emphasized.

When the moon passes through earth signs, root energy is enhanced. These are days for planting, transplanting, and harvesting root crops - for working with the below-ground, the hidden, the foundational. When the moon transits water signs, leaf energy is enhanced. Plant leafy greens, harvest leaves, attend to the foliage that captures light and breathes for the plant. When the moon moves through air signs, flower energy is enhanced. Work with blossoms, plant flowering plants, attend to pollination and beauty. When the moon traverses fire signs, fruit and seed energy is enhanced. Plant fruiting crops, harvest seeds and fruits, work with what the plant produces for reproduction.

This creates a rhythm within the lunar month - every month offers several root days, leaf days, flower days, and fruit days, woven together by the moon's journey through the zodiac. Biodynamic calendars translate these astronomical movements into practical guidance, offering a daily framework for attuning farm and garden work to celestial patterns.

Does it work? The question itself may miss the point. Biodynamic practitioners tend to be deeply attentive to their plants, their soil, their environment. They observe closely. They work with intention. This attention and intention produce results regardless of whether the specific astrological correspondences reflect "real" cosmic influences. And perhaps the distinction between "real" influence and the influence of heightened attention isn't as meaningful as we assume. Perhaps the cosmos works through us as much as on us - our attention becoming the mechanism through which celestial patterns shape earthly growth.

You don't need to adopt biodynamics completely to learn from its central insight: that we live in a cosmos, not just on an earth, and that cosmic rhythms may matter for our work with plants. Experiment. Track what happens when you plant root vegetables on root days versus leaf days. Notice whether flower-day harvests feel different from root-day harvests. Let your own experience teach you what these frameworks offer.

MAKING MEDICINE BY THE MOON

If the moon influences plants, she may also influence what we make from them. Traditional herbalists often timed their medicine-making to lunar phases, believing that when a preparation was begun and completed affected its quality in ways beyond chemistry - that the moon's energy at the moment of beginning infused the medicine with a particular quality that would persist in the finished preparation.

Beginning a tincture at new moon means the extraction process unfolds through the waxing phase, building toward fullness as the moon builds toward full. There's a sympathetic magic here - as the moon draws toward visibility, the menstruum draws constituents from plant into liquid. As lunar energy increases, the medicine strengthens. By full moon, the extraction peaks. The following two weeks of waning allow integration, settling, the medicine finding its coherence as the moon returns to darkness.

Some traditional preparations were timed to complete specific lunar durations. A tincture begun at new moon and strained at the following new moon has traveled one complete lunar cycle - emerging from darkness, building through light, releasing through waning, returning to darkness transformed. This feels complete in a way that an arbitrary four-week maceration doesn't, even if the chemistry is similar.

Different timing serves different purposes. A preparation meant for building, strengthening, or increasing might be begun at new moon and strained at full moon - maximum waxing energy, no waning. A preparation meant for releasing, cleansing, or clearing might be begun at full moon and strained at new moon - the medicine made during the letting-go phase, infused with that quality.

Does the timing actually change the medicine? In ways chemistry could measure, probably not significantly. In subtler ways - the quality practitioners call "energy" or "spirit" - perhaps. What's certain is that lunar timing creates rhythm and structure for your practice. When you know you'll begin tinctures at new moon, you prepare. You gather what you need. The deadline focuses attention. The practice becomes ritual, repeated monthly, deepening your relationship with both the plants and the moon.

And perhaps the intention matters as much as the timing. Medicine made with attention to the moon is medicine made with attention, period. That attention - that presence, that care, that recognition of participating in something larger than the mechanical mixing of plant and liquid - may be what infuses the medicine with qualities that transcend chemistry.

THE ANCIENT PARTNERSHIP

The moon has been the earth's companion for over four billion years. Born from violence - a Mars-sized body colliding with the young earth, debris coalescing into our silver satellite - she has been shaping life here ever since. This is not spiritual teaching; this is geological fact. But fact and teaching are not opposites. Sometimes fact is the deepest teaching.

The tides are her most obvious gift - and gift is not too strong a word. The rhythmic flooding and draining of tidal zones may have provided crucial environments for life's transition from sea to land. In those liminal spaces, neither fully aquatic nor fully terrestrial, early organisms could adapt gradually to conditions on shore. Without the moon's pull creating tides, the jump from sea to land might never have happened. We may owe our existence as land creatures to the moon.

Less obviously, the moon stabilizes Earth's axial tilt. Without her gravitational anchor, our axis would wobble chaotically over millions of years, creating extreme climate swings that might have made complex life impossible. The stable seasons we've been exploring - the very wheel of the year that organizes this book - depend on the moon holding us steady in our orientation to the sun.

Life evolved under moonlight. Before fire, before electricity, the full moon was the brightest light in the nighttime world - bright enough to hunt by, to travel by, to find a mate by, to be found by predators by. Entire ecosystems organized around her presence or absence. Nocturnal hunters learned the phases. Prey animals knew when to hide. Corals spawn in synchronized masses triggered by moonlight. Sea turtles nest on lunar schedules. Moths navigate by her constant position. The night world evolved in relationship with the moon.

Humans, too. Our ancestors lived by fire and moonlight, their activities shaped by whether she illuminated the night or left it dark. Our hormones, our sleep, our fertility - all evolved under lunar influence, in bodies that knew no artificial light to mask her phases. We are lunar creatures who have forgotten the relationship, insulated from the night sky that shaped us.

When you step outside under the full moon, you're meeting the same presence that watched over your ancestors for countless generations, that shaped the evolution of your body and your instincts, that has been the earth's partner since before there was any life to notice. This meeting is always available. The moon rises whether you watch or not. But when you watch - when you let yourself feel the ancient connection - you remember something your bones already know. You come home to a relationship that has been waiting for you to notice it.

Entering the Rhythm

How do you begin? Start simply. Start with attention. Start with willingness to notice what you've been ignoring.

First, simply know where the moon is in her cycle. Check a calendar, use an app, or learn to read her phases directly by looking. A waxing moon is illuminated on the right side (in the northern hemisphere) and growing; a waning moon is illuminated on the left and shrinking. When the moon's face is dark, she's new. When she's round and bright, she's full. This is basic lunar literacy - knowing, without having to look anything up, what phase the moon wears today.

Then, begin tracking correlations in your own experience. A simple log - moon phase and how you slept, how you feel, what you notice. Don't expect instant patterns; one month means nothing. Track for several months, preferably a year. Let the patterns reveal themselves. Your body may know things about lunar influence that your mind hasn't noticed yet.

Experiment in your herbal practice. Harvest the same plant at different phases and compare. Begin tinctures at new moon for several cycles, then try full moon starts, and notice if you perceive differences. Plant seeds at different phases and observe germination and growth. Your garden is an altar, your medicine-making a form of divination - ways of asking questions and receiving answers from a world that speaks, if you know how to listen.

Don't become rigid. The point is not to add rules that burden your life with guilt when you can't follow them. A plant harvested under the "wrong" moon is still medicine. A tincture begun whenever you got around to it still works. Lunar timing is an invitation into deeper relationship, not a test you pass or fail. Use it when you can. Release it when you can't. The moon will still be there tomorrow.

Let lunar awareness become a form of presence - a way of remembering, again and again, that you live in a cosmos. Each time you notice the moon, you step out of artificial time into something more real. Each time you align an activity with her rhythm, you choose participation over ignorance. This cumulative attention - not any single practice - is what shifts your experience of being alive.

EMBODIED PRACTICE: A LUNAR MONTH VIGIL

This practice invites you into a month of deliberate lunar attention - not as exercise but as vigil, a keeping of watch, an act of witness. Over one complete lunar cycle, you'll track the moon's journey, observe her reflections in your own body and life, and create a simple medicine timed to her rhythm. By the month's end, you'll have direct experience of what the moon offers when you turn toward her.

You'll need a way to track lunar phases. A simple journal for daily notes - just a sentence or two each day. The materials for making a small tincture: a jar, vodka or brandy, and a single herb you want to know more deeply. Nettle, chamomile, lemon balm, or calendula are good choices. And you'll need commitment to one month of attention, even when you don't feel like it, even when nothing seems to be happening.

Begin at new moon. If you're reading this at some other phase, wait. The waiting is your first practice - learning to align with rhythm rather than demanding rhythm conform to your schedule.

☽○☾ New Moon: The Beginning Before Beginning

On or within a day of the new moon, begin your vigil. If the sky is clear, go outside in the evening and stand in the darkness. The moon is there, invisible, her dark face turned toward you. Feel what this darkness feels like. Not empty - full of potential. Not absence - presence of another kind. This is the seed point, the moment before emergence.

In your journal, write the date and a few words about your state. Energy. Mood. Sleep quality. Body sensations. What's alive in your inner world. Keep it simple - you'll be doing this daily.

Today, begin your tincture. Place your chosen herb in a clean jar, filling it loosely about one-third full. Pour vodka or brandy over the herb until it's fully submerged with room to spare. Cap tightly. Label with the herb name, the date, and the words "new moon." As you prepare it, consider: this medicine will grow with the moon. What in you wants to grow alongside it? Set an intention - not a goal, but a direction of attention - for this coming cycle.

☽○☾ Waxing Moon: The Rising

For the next two weeks, maintain your daily practice. A few words in your journal noting the moon's phase and your own state. Look for the moon when you can - she rises later each day during the waxing phase, but she's present in afternoon and evening skies, growing brighter night by night.

Shake your tincture daily. This is not just mechanical mixing; it's tending, relationship, attention. As you shake, consider: what is being drawn out? What is building? The medicine strengthens as the moon strengthens. Notice if the tincture's color deepens. Notice how the herb is changing in the liquid.

Pay attention to your energy during this phase. Does it build as the moon builds? Do you feel more capable of initiative, more drawn to external engagement? Does sleep shift as full moon approaches? Let whatever you notice be information, not judgment. You're gathering data about your own lunar nature.

☽○☾ Full Moon: The Illumination

On the full moon, make time for deliberate presence with her. If the sky is clear, go outside and stand in the moonlight. Let it fall on your skin. Feel the difference from sunlight - silver rather than gold, cool rather than warm, reflected rather than direct. This light has traveled from the sun to the moon to you, transformed by the journey. The same light that has fallen on every generation of humans who ever lived, on every plant and creature, on all of earth for four billion years.

In your journal, record your state with particular attention. How did you sleep last night? How do you feel - energized, overwhelmed, restless, clear? Are emotions close to the surface? Let yourself feel whatever you feel without needing to explain it.

Your tincture is at its midpoint. The waxing phase has drawn out the plant's gifts; the waning phase will allow settling and integration. Shake it and hold it up to the moonlight if you can, letting the light pass through. What is this medicine becoming?

☽○☾ Waning Moon: The Returning

For the next two weeks, as the moon diminishes toward dark, continue your vigil. Your daily journal entries. Your daily shaking of the tincture. Your attention to where the moon is and what you notice in yourself.

Does your energy shift during the waning phase? Many people notice a turning inward, a pull toward completion and release, less available energy for external demands. The world may feel less receptive to effort; the inner world may feel more accessible. What is ready to be released in you as the moon releases her light?

As you approach the dark moon days before the next new moon, notice if energy ebbs to its lowest. Is there a call to rest? To slow down? To wait? This is the completion of the cycle, the return to the seed point, the pause before beginning again.

☽○☾ Second New Moon: Completion

On or near the new moon following your beginning - one complete lunar cycle - complete your vigil. Strain your tincture through cloth into a clean bottle. Squeeze the spent herb to release all liquid. Label with the herb name, the dates (new moon to new moon), and any words that feel true about what this medicine has become.

This is your first lunar-timed preparation - medicine that has traveled the full arc of a lunar month, beginning and ending in darkness, touching the full light between. Hold the bottle. Feel what it feels like to hold medicine made this way.

Read through your journal from the past month. What patterns do you notice? Did your experience differ between waxing and waning? How was full moon? How was dark moon? What surprised you? What confirmed what you already suspected? This review is part of the practice - making meaning from attention.

☽○☾ Continuing

One month is a beginning. Patterns that appear may not repeat; patterns that don't appear may emerge over several cycles. Continue tracking, in whatever form serves you, for at least several more months. A full year of lunar observation will teach you things a single month cannot.

Make more lunar-timed preparations. Experiment with beginning at different phases for different purposes. Let lunar awareness become part of how you practice herbalism, how you garden, how you understand your own rhythms.

What you're cultivating is not technique but relationship. The moon will continue her cycles whether you watch or not. But when you watch - when you make her rhythms part of your rhythm - you become more fully what you are: a creature of earth and sky, shaped by forces older than your species, participating in a dance you didn't invent but are always invited to join.

Reflection Questions

1. What has been your relationship with the moon? Has she been presence or backdrop, teacher or furniture?

2. Have you noticed correlations between lunar phases and your own experience - sleep, energy, mood, cycle? What might you discover if you started looking?

3. How do you hold the relationship between scientific knowing and intuitive knowing? Can both be true?

4. What calls you about working with lunar rhythms? What resistances arise?

5. What might it mean for your sense of place in the cosmos to take the moon seriously as influence, as teacher, as presence?

6. When you imagine yourself in relationship with the moon - not just knowing about her phases, but knowing her - what do you feel?

The moon has been teaching since before there were students.
She asks nothing but your attention.
Give it, and see what she offers in return.

Part Three
Becoming the Alchemist

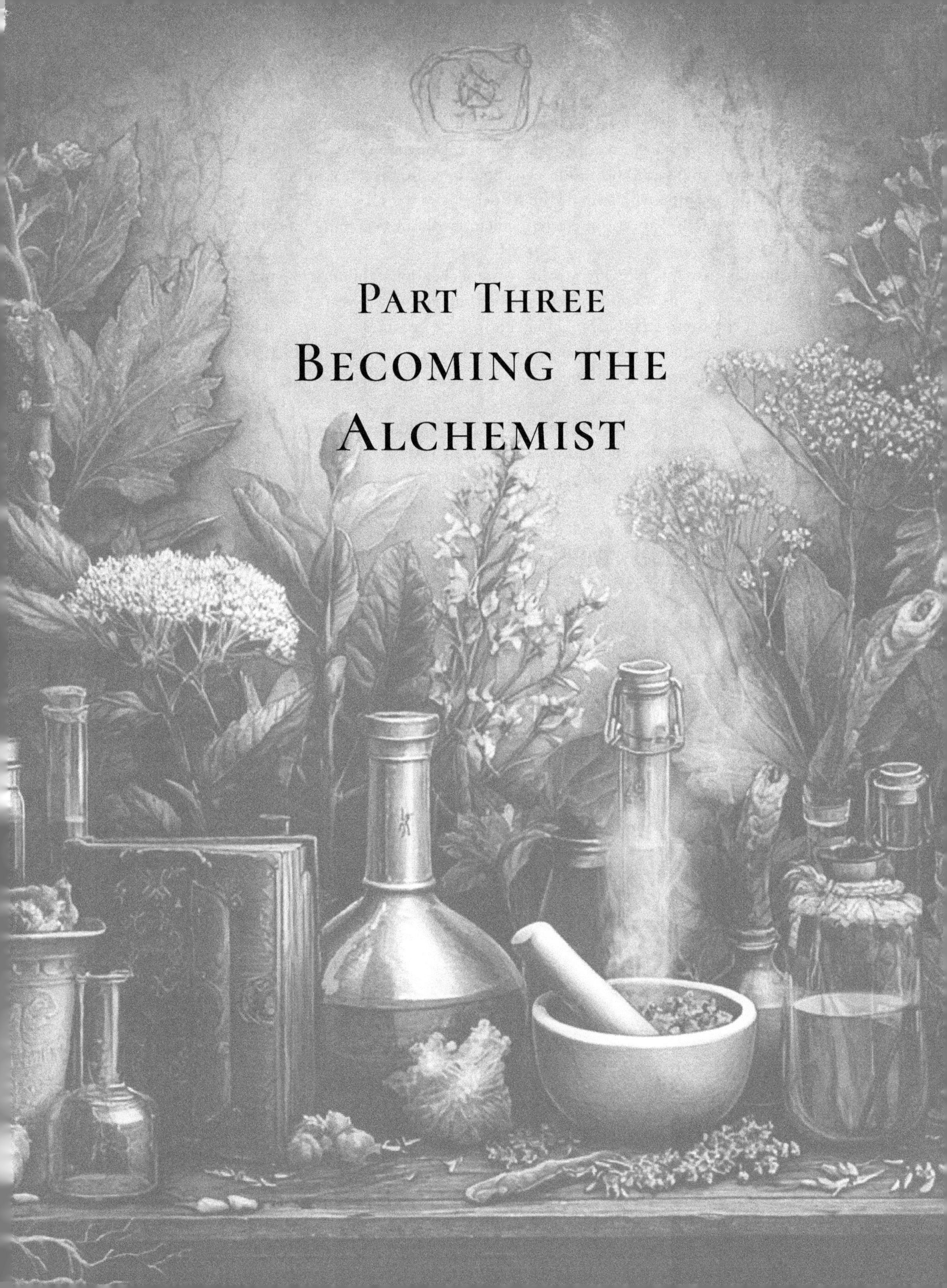

The alchemists of old sought to transform base metal into gold. This was never merely about chemistry - it was about transformation itself, about the possibility of elevating matter through understanding, intention, and sacred operation. The gold they sought was as much internal as external: the refinement of the practitioner alongside the refinement of the substance. You cannot transmute what you do not understand. You cannot create medicine without becoming, in some measure, medicinal yourself.

The chapters that follow invite you into the alchemist's laboratory - not as a sterile space of measurement and control, but as a vessel of transformation where you and the plants and the person seeking healing enter into relationship. Here, knowledge becomes art. Here, individual herbs become complex remedies tailored to the unique pattern of the person before you. Here, you learn to read not just symptoms but stories, not just bodies but souls, not just what is wrong but what is asking to be made right.

Alchemy has always operated on multiple levels simultaneously. The *prima materia* - the raw material - exists both outside and inside: the herbs in your apothecary, yes, but also the unrefined understanding you bring to the work. The *opus* - the great work - transforms both substance and practitioner. The *philosopher's stone* that catalyzes transformation is not separate from the one who wields it. As you learn to create formulas, you are also being created. As you learn to read patterns in others, you learn to read the patterns in yourself. As you offer medicine, you become medicine.

This is not clinical practice in the modern sense - detached, standardized, impersonal. This is the ancient art of the healer who knows that every encounter is unique, that every formula must be created fresh from the meeting of this plant intelligence with this human need in this moment. Protocols and guidelines serve as foundations, but the living work happens in the space between - in the intuition informed by knowledge, the creativity constrained by wisdom, the art that emerges when you have studied enough to trust what arises.

To become an alchemist is to accept a particular kind of responsibility: to be a vessel through which transformation can occur, while remaining humble about how much you do and don't understand. The plants are the true teachers. The body's wisdom is the true healer. You are the one who creates conditions, who facilitates meeting, who midwifes the transformation that wants to happen. This is enough. This is everything.

Chapter 10

The Art of Formulation

The Alchemist's Art

You have spent time with individual plants - learning their characters, their affinities, their gifts and cautions. You have explored the body's systems - the rivers and pathways through which life force moves. You have begun to recognize tissue states - the patterns of excess and deficiency, heat and cold, tension and laxity that reveal how a body has lost its balance. Now comes the art that weaves these threads together: formulation, the creation of complex remedies from the meeting of multiple plant intelligences with the unique pattern of the person before you.

This is where herbalism becomes truly alchemical. A single herb is powerful - a whole being offering its gifts. But a formula is something more: a community of plants, each bringing their particular medicine, arranged in relationship so that the whole becomes greater than the sum of its parts. The interaction between herbs creates something new, something that didn't exist in any individual plant. This is the mystery of combination, the alchemy of relationship.

Formulation cannot be reduced to protocol, though protocols can serve as training wheels while you develop your art. It cannot be standardized, though traditional frameworks offer maps for the territory. It requires both knowledge and intuition, both study and direct relationship with the plants, both humility about what you don't know and courage to create nonetheless. It is the difference between knowing recipes and knowing how to cook - the living skill that emerges only through practice, through mistakes, through the feedback loop of creating remedies and observing their effects.

Every formula you create is an experiment, a question asked of the plants and the body. Some will succeed beautifully. Some will miss. Some will teach you things no book could teach. This is the path of the alchemist - not certainty but engagement, not perfection but refinement, not knowing everything but being willing to learn from everything.

Why Create Formulas?

Single herbs are complete medicines - whole beings whose complexity we barely understand, offering effects that often surpass what we expect from their known constituents. There's nothing wrong with giving someone chamomile for their digestive distress and leaving it at that. Simplicity has its own power, its own clarity.

But human beings are not simple. They rarely come to you with a single issue in a single system. The woman with digestive problems is also anxious. The anxiety is disrupting her sleep. The poor sleep is affecting her hormones. The hormonal imbalance is making the digestive issues worse. Where do you begin? Which thread do you pull?

Formulas allow you to address this complexity - to work with multiple aspects of a pattern simultaneously, to support several body systems at once, to match the medicine to the actual human rather than to a simplified version of their complaint. A well-constructed formula might calm the nervous system while supporting digestion while balancing hormones while improving sleep - not by including a different herb for each issue, but by choosing herbs whose actions overlap and reinforce each other, creating a web of support that addresses the whole pattern.

Formulas also allow you to balance energetics. If someone needs a strongly cooling herb for inflammation but runs constitutionally cold, you can include warming herbs that prevent the formula from chilling them further. If a sedating herb is needed for sleep but the person also struggles with morning fatigue, you can add herbs that prevent excessive heaviness. The formula becomes a balanced whole, appropriate for this person rather than just for this condition.

And formulas create synergy - interactions between herbs that produce effects beyond what any herb could produce alone. Some herbs enhance the absorption of others. Some potentiate each other's actions. Some moderate each other's side effects. The traditional formulas that have survived centuries of use often contain this embedded wisdom - combinations that work better together than theory would predict, refined by generations of observation.

Consider the difference. For someone whose digestive distress is rooted in stress: a single herb approach might offer chamomile - digestive and calming, a good choice. But a formula might offer chamomile for its digestive and calming gifts, lemon balm to lift the spirits and support the gut-brain connection, fennel to release trapped gas and ease cramping, a small amount of ginger to warm the digestion and activate the formula, and bitters to stimulate the digestive secretions that stress has suppressed. This formula addresses not just the symptom but the pattern - the stress, the stagnation, the dampened digestive fire, the trapped wind, the depleted secretions. It meets the person where they actually are.

Traditional Frameworks: Maps for the Territory

Traditional medicine systems developed sophisticated approaches to formula construction over centuries of collective observation. These frameworks are not rules to follow blindly but maps that can orient you in complex territory - scaffolding that supports your own developing art until you internalize the principles deeply enough to work from them intuitively.

The Chinese Medicine model of formula construction is particularly elegant and adaptable. It conceives of herbs playing different roles within a formula, like musicians in an ensemble or members of a council - each with a specific function, arranged in relationship to create a coherent whole.

The Council of Herbs

The Sovereign - sometimes called the Chief or King - is the primary herb addressing the main complaint. This is the heart of the formula, the herb whose action most directly targets what needs to change. In a formula for anxiety with insomnia, the sovereign might be passionflower - powerfully anxiolytic and sleep-promoting, capable of shifting the pattern on its own. The sovereign typically comprises the largest proportion of the formula, because it's doing the primary work.

The Minister - sometimes called the Deputy - supports the sovereign's action and addresses secondary aspects of the pattern. If passionflower is sovereign for anxiety with insomnia, skullcap might serve as minister - also calming, also supportive of sleep, but with particular affinity for the racing, circular thoughts that keep the mind from settling. The minister reinforces and extends the sovereign's work.

The Assistant -fills several possible roles: moderating any harsh effects of stronger herbs, harmonizing the formula's overall energetics, addressing additional symptoms, or balancing the blend to make it appropriate for the specific person. In the anxiety formula, chamomile might serve as assistant - gentle, harmonizing, supportive of digestion (since anxiety often disrupts the gut), preventing the formula from being too heavily sedating. Lemon balm might also serve as assistant, adding its uplifting quality to balance the downward, sleep-promoting thrust of the other herbs.

The Messenger - sometimes called the Envoy or Guide - directs the formula to its target, enhances absorption and circulation, or harmonizes the entire blend. A small amount of ginger often serves this role: warming, activating, helping the other herbs reach where they're needed, supporting digestion so the medicine is well-absorbed. The messenger is typically a small proportion of the formula - a catalyst, not a main ingredient.

Not every formula needs all four roles. Simple formulas might have only a sovereign and minister. Complex patterns might call for multiple assistants. The framework is not a requirement but a way of thinking - a lens that helps you consider what each herb is contributing and whether the formula as a whole is coherent and complete.

The Energetic Equation

Every herb carries energetic qualities - warming or cooling, drying or moistening, stimulating or sedating, lifting or grounding. Every person has their own energetic pattern - constitutional tendencies toward heat or cold, dampness or dryness, excess or deficiency. The art of formulation includes matching the formula's overall energetics to what the person actually needs.

This sounds simple but requires attention. If someone has inflammation - a heat pattern - they likely need cooling herbs. But if they're also constitutionally cold (always chilled, cold hands and feet, craving warm foods), a strongly cooling formula might suppress the inflammation while making them feel worse overall. The art is finding the balance: enough cooling to address the heat pattern, enough warming to not overwhelm a cold constitution.

Consider a formula for digestive inflammation. The primary herbs might be cooling and soothing - marshmallow root to coat and protect inflamed tissue, calendula to reduce inflammation and support healing, chamomile to calm both gut and nervous system. These are all cooling herbs, appropriate for a heat condition. But adding a small amount of warming ginger prevents the formula from being too cold, activates digestion (which cold can dampen), and helps the other herbs circulate where they're needed. The overall formula is cooling, matching the condition, but not so cold that it creates new imbalances.

The same thinking applies to other energetic qualities. A formula for dry, irritated tissue needs moistening herbs - but too much moistening can create stagnation, so you might include something mildly moving. A formula for someone with excess might need draining or clearing herbs - but including some nourishing support prevents depleting them further. Every formula is a balance, an equation that must account for the condition being addressed *and* the person experiencing it.

Learn to feel into the formula you're creating. Does it feel balanced? Does it feel appropriate for this person? Sometimes your intuition will register something off before your analytical mind can identify what it is. Trust that registration. Investigate it. The formula is a living thing you're bringing into being - develop relationship with it, not just analysis of it.

Creating a Formula: The Living Process

There's no single right way to create a formula, but there's a natural movement from understanding to creation that most experienced formulators follow, whether they articulate it this way or not. This is not a checklist to complete mechanically but a dance to learn through repetition until it becomes second nature.

First: Listen

Before you can create medicine for someone, you must understand what they need. This requires listening - not just to words but to patterns, not just to complaints but to the story underneath the complaints. What are their primary concerns? What symptoms do they describe, and what do those symptoms suggest about underlying imbalances? What's their constitution - do they tend toward heat or cold, dampness or dryness, excess or deficiency? What body systems seem involved? What has their journey been - how long has this pattern existed, what has made it better or worse, what have they already tried?

This listening is also observation. What do you notice about them that they haven't told you? Their energy, their color, their voice, how they hold their body, what they emphasize and what they avoid? Every person is a text to be read, a pattern to be perceived. Some of this perception will be conscious analysis; some will be intuitive registration that you can't fully articulate but can learn to trust.

And this listening includes what they don't say but what your knowledge suggests you should ask.

Are there contraindications you need to rule out? Medications that might interact? Conditions that require medical care rather than herbal support? Pregnancy? The questions you ask shape what you learn; learn to ask the questions that matter.

Second: Understand

From listening emerges understanding - your assessment of what's actually happening beneath the surface symptoms. What tissue states are present? What patterns can you name? What seems like root cause and what seems like downstream effect? Where is the body's wisdom struggling, and what support might help?

This is where your study of body systems and tissue states and herbal energetics comes to life. You're not just collecting symptoms; you're reading a pattern. The headaches and digestive issues and irritability might all be expressions of a single underlying liver congestion. The fatigue and recurrent infections and slow healing might all point to immune depletion. The multiple unrelated complaints might be stress expressing through every available channel. Your understanding shapes what you'll address.

This understanding also includes what you *cannot* understand - the limits of your assessment, the possibilities you can't rule out, the uncertainty inherent in working with complex human beings. Humility belongs here. You're not diagnosing disease; you're reading patterns. You're not certain; you're creating a working hypothesis that your formula will test.

Third: Envision

Before reaching for specific herbs, get clear on what you're trying to accomplish. What needs to change? What needs support? What's the direction of movement you're trying to facilitate? Are you trying to cool heat, warm cold, dry dampness, moisten dryness, stimulate deficiency, calm excess, release tension, build reserves? Get clear on the therapeutic direction before choosing the vehicles that will travel it.

This visioning might include multiple goals, prioritized by importance. For the perimenopausal woman with hot flashes, irritability, sleep disruption, and breast tenderness, the therapeutic goals might be: primarily, cool the heat pattern (hot flashes, night sweats); secondarily, support the nervous system (irritability, sleep); tertiarily, address the liver component (breast tenderness suggests liver involvement). Knowing the priorities helps you choose your sovereign and organize your supporting cast.

Fourth: Choose

Now you select the herbs - the specific plants whose medicine will meet this person's need. Start with the sovereign: what herb most directly addresses the primary therapeutic goal with energetics appropriate for this person? For hot flashes with heat signs, black cohosh might be sovereign - cooling, specific for menopausal heat, well-studied for this use.

Then the minister: what supports and extends the sovereign's action while addressing secondary aspects? Sage might serve here - also cooling, specifically reduces sweating, addresses hot flashes from a different angle. Motherwort might join - calming for the irritability and anxiety, specific for menopausal transition, supportive of the heart that often races with hot flashes.

Then assistants: what balances, harmonizes, addresses remaining concerns? Skullcap for the sleep disruption and nervous system support. Dandelion root for gentle liver support, addressing that breast tenderness and helping the body process the hormonal shifts. Licorice in small amount to harmonize the formula and support the adrenal glands that are working hard during this transition.

As you choose, you're constantly checking: Do these herbs work together? Are the energetics balanced and appropriate? Is anything missing? Is anything redundant? Does the formula address the whole pattern or just part of it?

Fifth: Evaluate

Before finalizing, step back and assess the formula as a whole. Check the energetics: is this formula appropriately cooling for a heat pattern? Is it too cold for someone who needs some warmth? Are there enough warming or activating herbs to prevent stagnation?

Check for safety: are there any contraindications given this person's situation? Any potential interactions between herbs, or between herbs and medications? Anything that gives you pause?

Check for coherence: does the formula feel like a unified whole, or like a random collection of potentially useful herbs? Can you articulate what each herb is contributing and why it belongs?

And check for practicality: will the person actually take this? Is the form appropriate (tincture, tea, capsule)? Is the taste acceptable? Is the cost manageable? Is the dosing schedule realistic for their life? A perfect formula that sits unused is worse than a good-enough formula that they take consistently.

Reading the Story: The Alchemist's Assessment

Every person who comes to you seeking herbal support is a story in progress - a pattern unfolding over time, a body adapting to circumstances, a life seeking balance. Your role is to read this story well enough to offer medicine that serves it. This reading has both art and structure to it.

The structure: you're gathering information on several levels. First, their subjective experience - what they tell you about their symptoms, their concerns, their history, what makes things better or worse. This is their story in their words, valuable for what it reveals and also for what it emphasizes, avoids, or doesn't notice.

Second, your objective observations - what you notice directly. This might include formal assessments if you're trained in them (tongue and pulse reading, for instance), but it also includes simple observation: their energy, their color, their voice quality, how they sit and move, what their skin and eyes and nails tell you, what you sense in the room when you're with them. Some of this you can articulate; some you register without being able to name it.

Third, your assessment - your synthesis of what you've heard and observed into a working understanding of the pattern. What tissue states are present? What seems to be the root? What's the constitutional picture? This is your clinical thinking made explicit, the story as you understand it.

Fourth, your plan - the formula you'll create, the dosing you'll recommend, the lifestyle suggestions that support the herbal work, the timeline for follow-up, the conditions under which they should seek other care. This is your response to the story, your offer of medicine for this moment in their journey.

Recording these four elements - subjective, objective, assessment, plan - creates documentation you can return to, learn from, and build on. It allows you to track what you offered and what resulted. Over time, your documentation becomes a record of your developing art, a text you can study to refine your practice.

But don't let structure eclipse art. The person before you is not a form to fill out. They're a living mystery, partially knowable, always more than your assessment can capture. Hold your understanding loosely. Be willing to be surprised. The best practitioners combine rigor with receptivity - structured thinking that stays open to what doesn't fit the structure.

An Example: Reading and Responding

Let's walk through a formulation process, not as template to copy but as illustration of how these principles come together in practice.

The person: A woman in her early forties, in the perimenopausal transition. She comes seeking support for hot flashes that wake her at night, leaving her sleep-deprived and irritable. She mentions breast tenderness before her period, which has become irregular - sometimes coming every three weeks, sometimes skipping. Her mood feels unstable; she describes herself as "not herself," easily overwhelmed by things she used to handle easily.

What you observe: She speaks quickly, seems somewhat agitated, makes good eye contact but with an intensity that suggests tension. Her complexion has reddish undertones. She mentions she's been craving sweets and drinking more coffee to get through the exhausted days.

Your assessment: A heat pattern is clear - the hot flashes, night sweats, reddish complexion, agitation. The irritability and breast tenderness suggest liver involvement; in traditional terms, liver heat or liver qi stagnation generating heat. The nervous system is affected - both from the hormonal shifts and from the sleep deprivation. The irregular cycles confirm perimenopausal transition. The sugar cravings and increased coffee suggest she's running on stress hormones, depleting herself further.

Therapeutic goals: Cool the heat pattern (hot flashes, night sweats). Support the liver in this transition. Calm and restore the nervous system. Improve sleep. Help her body adapt to the hormonal shifts of perimenopause.

The formula:

- Black cohosh serves as sovereign - cooling, specific for hot flashes, well-matched to her heat pattern, supported by considerable research for menopausal symptoms. Two parts.
- Sage joins as minister - also cooling, specifically reduces sweating, addresses the night

sweats from a different angle than black cohosh, traditional for menopausal heat. One and a half parts.
- Motherwort as second minister - calming for the anxiety and irritability, specific for heart symptoms that often accompany hot flashes (racing, palpitations), has affinity for the uterus and the menopausal transition. One and a half parts.
- Skullcap as assistant - nervine support for the irritability and sleep disruption, cooling, specific for the racing mind that can prevent sleep. One part.
- Dandelion root as assistant - gentle liver support for the breast tenderness and irritability, helping the body process the hormonal shifts, not adding heat. One part.
- Licorice as harmonizer - small amount to unify the formula, support the adrenals, add a touch of sweetness that improves compliance. Half part.

Energetic check: The formula is predominantly cooling - appropriate for her heat pattern. Nothing excessively heating. The cooling is balanced enough that it shouldn't chill her. The formula addresses hormonal transition, nervous system, liver, and sleep. No evident contraindications for her situation.

Preparation and dosing: Tincture blend, for convenience and consistent dosing. Four to five milliliters two to three times daily. Review in four to six weeks.

Additional support: Suggest reducing coffee (which aggravates heat and depletes her further) and sugar (which feeds the cycle of depletion). Encourage earlier bedtime to catch whatever sleep is possible. Cool, bitter foods might help - salads, bitter greens. Deep breathing when hot flashes begin can sometimes reduce their intensity.

This is one formula, created for one person at one moment in time. Another person with similar complaints but different constitution might need different herbs. The same person at a different stage of her transition might need a different formula. This is the art: matching the medicine to the moment.

The Wisdom of Simplicity

Not every situation calls for complex formulation. Sometimes a single herb is exactly right - well-matched to the need, sufficient on its own, elegant in its simplicity. Sometimes a simple formula of two or three herbs addresses the pattern without unnecessary complexity. The goal is appropriate response, not impressive complexity.

Use single herbs when the issue is straightforward and a specific herb is clearly indicated. When chamomile is perfect for this moment, give chamomile. Don't add other herbs just to have a formula. Single herbs also allow you to learn how that plant works in practice - what it does for this person, how they respond, what you can observe. Before you combine, know the individuals.

Use simple formulas of two or three herbs when the pattern has a clear primary cause with perhaps a secondary element - when you can address what's needed without elaborate construction. Simple formulas are also appropriate for people who are sensitive or reactive, where multiple herbs might overwhelm. And they allow clearer observation of effects; if something isn't working, you know more easily what to adjust.

Use complex formulas of four to seven herbs when the pattern is truly complex - multiple body systems involved, constitutional factors requiring balance, chronic conditions with many facets. Complex formulas serve genuine complexity, not the desire to seem sophisticated.

More herbs is not better. Elegant simplicity is often most effective. Each herb you add should earn its place in the formula - contributing something specific that the formula needs and would lack without it. If you can't articulate why an herb belongs, it probably doesn't.

Common Patterns: Starting Points for Adaptation

Over time, you'll develop familiarity with formulas that work well for common patterns. These are not protocols to apply mindlessly but starting points to adapt - familiar frameworks you modify for the specific person before you. Here are a few examples to illustrate the form.

A Digestive Bitters Formula

For weak or sluggish digestion - the kind where food sits heavy, where there's bloating and gas, where the body seems to have forgotten how to process what it receives. Dandelion root or gentian as sovereign, waking the bitter receptors that trigger digestive secretions. Yellow dock or burdock as minister, supporting liver function and gentle elimination. Chamomile or fennel as assistant, soothing and carminative. Ginger or orange peel as messenger, warming and activating. The proportions and specific herbs shift based on whether the person runs hot or cold, whether constipation or loose stool accompanies, whether there's anxiety or calm, but the form remains: bitters awakening digestion, support for processing, something to ease discomfort, something to warm and move.

A Sleep Formula

For the mind that won't quiet, the body that won't settle, the sleep that won't come or won't stay. Passionflower or valerian as sovereign, depending on whether the pattern is more anxious (passionflower) or more simply wakeful (valerian). Skullcap as minister, calming the specific pattern of racing thoughts. Chamomile and lavender as assistants, gentling the formula, supporting the body's own movement toward rest. Lemon balm or catnip as messenger/harmonizer, uplifting slightly to prevent heavy morning fog. The formula changes based on what's preventing sleep - anxiety, pain, restless legs, night waking, difficulty falling asleep versus staying asleep - but the form provides a starting point.

A Nervous System Restoration Formula

For the depleted, burned-out nervous system - the one that has been running on stress hormones for too long and has lost its resilience. Milky oats as sovereign, the supreme nervous system restorative, rebuilding what has been exhausted. Ashwagandha as minister, adaptogenic and calming, helping the body recover its capacity to handle stress. Skullcap as assistant, addressing the specific pattern of overwrought thinking, both calming and tonic. Nettles as assistant, providing mineral nourishment for the physical substrate. Licorice or ginger as harmonizer, unifying and activating. This formula isn't for acute anxiety; it's for the long, slow rebuilding after prolonged depletion.

Safety: The Alchemist's Responsibility

With the power to create medicine comes responsibility to do so safely. The alchemist who harms through ignorance or carelessness has betrayed the art. Safety consciousness should be woven through every step of your formulation process, not added as an afterthought.

For each herb you consider, know its contraindications. Know who shouldn't take it - pregnancy, nursing, specific medical conditions, medications. Know its potential adverse effects and how to recognize them. This knowledge should be automatic, part of how you hold the herb in your mind.

Consider interactions - between the herbs in your formula and between your formula and any medications the person takes. Some interactions are well-documented (St. John's wort and many pharmaceuticals). Others are theoretical but worth caution (combining multiple anticoagulant herbs, for instance). When you're uncertain, err on the side of caution. Consult references. Ask colleagues with more experience. Work with the person's healthcare providers when appropriate.

Match the energetics appropriately. A strongly cooling formula for someone who runs cold can cause harm. A strongly heating formula for someone with heat signs can aggravate. The formula needs to fit the person, not just the condition.

Start with lower doses when you're unsure, especially for sensitive individuals or when using herbs you haven't used before. You can always increase; you can't take back what you've given. Monitor carefully. Ask about effects at follow-up - not just whether the primary complaint improved but whether anything unexpected or concerning occurred.

And know the limits of herbal support. Some conditions require medical care. Some symptoms suggest pathology that needs diagnosis. Some situations are emergencies. Part of safety is knowing when to refer, when to insist on medical evaluation, when herbal support is not enough. The ego that wants to help should never override the wisdom that recognizes limits.

Scope and Humility

The alchemist works within bounds - not because the art is limited but because wisdom requires knowing what you can and cannot do. Understanding your scope of practice is not a legal technicality; it's a form of integrity.

What you can do: read patterns in the body, assess tissue states and constitutional factors, recommend herbs and formulas matched to what you observe, educate about plant medicine, support lifestyle changes that serve health, encourage self-care and body wisdom, work alongside medical care as a complementary support.

What you cannot do: diagnose disease (that's the province of licensed medical professionals), prescribe pharmaceuticals, perform medical procedures, promise cures or make claims you can't support, replace necessary medical care, practice beyond the limits of your training and competence.

This distinction matters. When someone comes with symptoms that might indicate serious pathology, you refer for diagnosis. When someone needs medical treatment, you support them in getting it - not compete with it. When something is beyond your training, you say so honestly. Humility is not weakness; it's wisdom. The ego that needs to have all the answers serves no one.

The best herbal practitioners collaborate beautifully with medical care. They fill gaps that medicine doesn't fill. They support people before they need medical intervention and after, when they're recovering. They offer what plants offer - which is much - without claiming to offer what only medicine can offer. This collaboration serves people better than either approach alone.

And the deepest humility: the plants are the healers, not you. The body's wisdom is what heals, not your formula. You are a facilitator, a matchmaker, a creator of conditions. This is enough. This is the true alchemist's position - powerful in what you can offer, humble about the mystery you serve.

Developing Your Own Alchemical Style

Every alchemist eventually develops their own way of working - a style shaped by training, by the traditions that resonate, by the plants that become allies, by the people they serve, by temperament and philosophy. This style is not something to force or choose prematurely; it emerges through practice, through the slow accumulation of experience that gradually reveals your particular gifts and inclinations.

Some practitioners lean toward energetic and constitutional approaches - reading the person's fundamental pattern and matching herbs primarily by energetics. Others emphasize research and evidence, wanting scientific support for their choices. Some work within traditional systems - Chinese medicine, Ayurveda, Western physiomedicalism - that provide complete frameworks. Others develop eclectic approaches that draw from multiple traditions. Some cultivate intuitive and spiritual dimensions of plant work. Some focus on bioregional practice, working primarily with plants from their local landscape.

Most effective practitioners blend multiple approaches: traditional wisdom that has survived centuries of testing, modern research that illuminates mechanisms and confirms (or challenges) tradition, direct relationship with plants through growing, harvesting, and preparing them, clinical observation of what actually works in practice, intuition developed through attention and refined by feedback, and humility that keeps learning central to the work.

Your style will emerge. Trust the process. Let your training and experience and the plants themselves shape you. Don't try to be something you're not, but also don't limit yourself to what feels comfortable. Growth requires stretching. Mastery requires time.

Embodied Practice: Creating Your First Formula

This practice invites you to create a formula - not for someone else, but for yourself. You are the person you know best, the one whose patterns you can read most directly, the one who can give you feedback on what your creation does. This is practice, not perfection. The goal is to move through the process, to feel how it works in your hands.

You'll need your apothecary - whatever herbs you have available in tincture form (if you want to make a tincture blend) or dried form (if you want to make a tea blend). You'll need a journal for recording your process. And you'll need honest self-reflection about what you actually need support with right now.

Listen to Yourself

Begin by sitting quietly and turning attention inward. What in you is asking for support right now? Not what you think you should work on, not what seems most serious, but what's actually calling for attention. It might be sleep, digestion, anxiety, energy, mood, immunity, hormones - or something more subtle that you'll need to name for yourself.

In your journal, write down your primary concern and any secondary aspects that seem related. Be specific: not just "sleep" but "difficulty falling asleep because my mind races" or "waking at 3am and not being able to get back to sleep."

Note your constitution as you understand it. Do you run hot or cold? Dry or damp? Are you generally high energy or low? Do you tend toward excess or deficiency? What patterns do you notice in yourself?

Understand the Pattern

What tissue states might be present in what you're experiencing? What body systems seem involved? What does your training suggest about what's happening beneath the surface symptoms?

Write down your assessment. What's the pattern as you understand it? What seems like root cause versus symptom? What direction of change are you hoping to support - cooling, warming, calming, stimulating, moistening, drying, building, clearing?

Choose Your Herbs

Looking at what you have available, what herb might serve as sovereign - the primary herb addressing your main concern? It should have the right energetics for your constitution and the right actions for your pattern. Write down your choice and why.

What might serve as minister, supporting the sovereign and addressing secondary aspects? What as assistant, harmonizing and balancing? Do you need a messenger to activate and direct?

Choose your herbs - probably three to five for this practice. Write down each and its role in the formula. Note the proportions you'll use (the sovereign typically being the largest proportion).

Evaluate

Before blending, evaluate your formula. Are the energetics balanced and appropriate for your constitution? Do the herbs work well together? Are there any safety concerns for you personally (medications, conditions, sensitivities)? Does the formula address the pattern you identified?

Make any adjustments that seem needed. Then blend your formula - measuring tinctures into a bottle or mixing dried herbs in a container. Label clearly with contents, proportions, and date.

Take and Observe

Take your formula for at least two weeks, following appropriate dosing for the form you chose. Keep notes on what you observe - effects on your primary concern, any secondary effects, how you feel overall. Note what works and what doesn't, what you might adjust if you made this formula again.

This observation is where you learn. The formula is a question; your body's response is the answer. Pay attention. Let the feedback inform your developing art.

You have now created a formula. It may be brilliant or mediocre or somewhere between. What matters is that you've moved through the process, felt it in your hands, created something real that you can learn from. This is how the art develops - not by reading alone but by doing, by trying, by letting the work teach you.

Reflection Questions

1. What is your emerging approach to formulation? What feels natural, and what feels challenging?

2. How do you hold the relationship between structure (traditional frameworks, systematic thinking) and intuition in your practice?

3. What safety considerations feel most important to you? Where do you need to develop more knowledge?

4. How do you understand your scope of practice? Where are its boundaries, and how do you honor them?

. . .

5. What kind of alchemist are you becoming? What traditions, approaches, and relationships are shaping you?

6. What does it mean to you to be a vessel through which transformation can occur, rather than the source of transformation itself?

The formula is a vessel. You are a vessel.
What transforms is the meeting - plant and person, need and gift.
You are learning to create the conditions for transformation.

The Opus Complete

Chapter 11

The Opus Complete

The Threshold Crossed

When you began this journey, you stood at a threshold. Perhaps you looked at plants and saw ingredients, resources, green things to be used. Perhaps you knew already that they were more than this but didn't yet have the language or the relationship to know *how* much more. You came seeking knowledge, and knowledge you have gained. But something else has happened in the process - something the alchemists always knew would happen to those who truly engaged the work.

You have been transformed.

This is the secret at the heart of alchemy: the *opus* transforms the operator as surely as it transforms the substance. You cannot spend months in deep relationship with plants - learning their languages, tasting their essences, preparing their medicines, studying the bodies they heal - without being changed by the encounter. The knowledge has become part of you. But more than knowledge: a way of seeing, a way of being, a way of moving through the world that recognizes kinship where before you saw only separation.

Now you see teachers where you once saw weeds. You feel the pulse of the season in your own body. You read the signs that tissues offer. You understand that healing is not something you do to bodies but something you facilitate between plant intelligence and body wisdom. You have developed the clinical thinking to create formulas from relationship, matching the specificity of the plant to the specificity of the person. You have walked through the wheel of the year, learning spring's clearing and summer's vitality and autumn's gathering and winter's deep rest. You have followed the moon through her phases. You have begun to sense yourself as part of something vast and ancient and alive.

This is not just information you have acquired. This is who you have become.

The alchemists had a name for this moment: the *rubedo*, the reddening, the final stage of the great work when what was separated reunites, when what was transformed emerges in its new form. The *nigredo* of unknowing, the *albedo* of purification through study, the *citrinitas* of dawning understanding - all these have led here, to the completion that is also a beginning. The gold emerges from the crucible. The philosopher's stone forms. The medicine is made.

You are the alchemist.

The Weaving Complete

You have learned many things - perhaps more than you can easily hold in mind at once. There were the foundational teachings: reciprocal relationship with plants as the ground from which everything else grows, energetics as the language through which plants and bodies speak, preparation methods as alchemical processes that transform crude plant matter into refined medicine. There was the bridge into clinical thinking: reading tissue states, recognizing patterns, learning to match plant to person with increasing sophistication.

There was the journey through the seasons - spring's rising energy with its support for digestion, liver, lymphatic clearing; summer's full expression with its care for respiratory, immune, and cardiovascular vitality; autumn's gathering with its nourishment of nervous system and bones; winter's deep rest with its attention to reproductive health and the restoration that only stillness can bring. There was the lunar thread woven through it all, the celestial rhythm that patterns plant and body alike. And there was the art of formulation - learning to combine individual plant allies into complex medicines that address the whole person.

Integration means seeing how all these pieces connect - not as separate topics you studied but as facets of a single understanding, a unified way of seeing and working. The energetics you learned early inform the formulas you create now. The tissue states you learned to read connect to the body systems you studied in detail. The seasonal wisdom you absorbed shapes when and how you harvest, prepare, and prescribe. The reciprocity that grounded you at the beginning deepens as you practice, becoming not just philosophy but lived relationship.

Take time to see these connections. Review what you have learned, not as memorization but as contemplation. How does spring's liver support connect to autumn's nervous system nourishment, when the liver's congestion so often manifests as irritability and tension? How does winter's reproductive wisdom connect to summer's cardiovascular support, when hormones and heart are so intimately related? How do the adaptogens that span seasons relate to the nervines that specific seasons emphasize?

The knowledge is not separate pieces filed in separate compartments. It is a living whole, a web where every thread connects to every other thread. Your understanding becomes truly integrated when you can move fluidly between these connections, drawing on whatever is relevant to the person and pattern before you.

Your Living Materia Medica

By now, you should have detailed profiles for dozens of herbs - fifty or more, if you have been diligent. But "profiles" does not quite capture what you have built. You have built relationships, documented in the form of profiles. Each entry in your materia medica represents a plant you have met, tasted, prepared, studied, worked with. Each contains your direct sensory experience - what you tasted, what you felt, what you observed in yourself and others. Each holds the clinical thinking you have developed - when and how and for whom you would use this plant. Each carries the relationship you have built.

This is *your* materia medica, distinct from any book or reference you might consult. It holds your knowledge, your experience, your relationships. It is a living document that will grow throughout your practice - every herb you study, every observation you make, every person you work with adding to what you know and deepening what you understand.

Review what you have built. Notice which herbs you feel most confident with - these are your core allies, the plants you can reach for with certainty. Notice which herbs call to you most strongly, which ones you feel drawn to learn more deeply - these may be your specialist herbs, the plants through whom you develop particular expertise. Notice which body systems you understand best and which remain more mysterious - this tells you where to focus continued study.

Notice too how your understanding has deepened over time. The herbs you met early in your journey - do you know them differently now than you did then? Has your relationship with them grown as you've grown? Return to those early profiles and add what you now know. Let your materia medica be truly living, updated and expanded with every season of practice.

And continue adding. Every herb you study from here forward, every clinical observation, every piece of research that changes your understanding, every seasonal variation you notice - add it to your materia medica. This document will become, over years of practice, a treasure of accumulated wisdom. It will be your own book of plant medicine, written from your own relationship with the green world.

THE SKILLS YOU HAVE DEVELOPED

Beyond the herbs themselves, you have developed capacities - ways of thinking and perceiving and assessing that are distinct from knowledge of any particular plant. You can now observe tissue states, reading the signs that bodies offer about their patterns of imbalance. You can ask the questions that reveal underlying patterns, listening for what people say and don't say, noticing what they emphasize and what they avoid. You can think energetically - recognizing hot and cold, dry and damp, excess and deficiency - and match your recommendations to what you perceive.

You understand when a single herb is appropriate and when a formula better serves, and you can create formulas that address complex patterns with coherent, balanced combinations. You can document your work in ways that support your own learning and meet professional standards. You know your scope - what you can appropriately offer and where the boundaries lie - and you know when to refer, when to collaborate, when to step back and let other practitioners lead.

These skills will deepen with every person you work with. Each consultation teaches you something - about herbs, about bodies, about the patterns of human suffering and the pathways toward balance. Each formula you create refines your thinking about combination and proportion and energetic balance. Each herb you use builds relationship with that plant, revealing aspects that study alone could not reveal. Each mistake - and there will be mistakes - teaches you something valuable if you're willing to learn from it.

You complete this book not as an expert but as a skilled beginner - which is exactly where you should be. You have solid foundation, clinical thinking skills, direct relationships with medicinal plants, ability to create effective formulas, understanding of your scope and ethics, tools to continue learning. What you don't yet have is the accumulated experience that turns foundation into mastery. That comes only through practice, through years of showing up and doing the work and learning from what happens.

Trust the process. You know enough to begin. Beginning is how you learn the rest.

Your Unique Path

What kind of herbalist are you becoming? The question is not rhetorical. There are many ways to walk this path, and finding yours is part of the work ahead.

Some herbalists focus on clinical practice - seeing clients individually or in groups, creating custom formulas, providing consultations that address the whole person. The clinical herbalist becomes skilled at reading patterns and matching plants to people, developing relationships with clients over time, witnessing the transformations that herbal medicine can support.

Some herbalists orient toward community - teaching classes and workshops, making medicine available to those who couldn't otherwise access it, focusing on accessible and affordable herbalism that serves those most in need. The community herbalist builds local plant knowledge, passes on skills, creates resilience at the neighborhood and bioregional level.

Some herbalists become medicine makers - crafting tinctures and salves and teas and elixirs with the care of true artisans, sharing plant medicine through farmers' markets or apothecary shops or online offerings. The medicine maker develops deep skill in preparation methods, sources herbs ethically and sustainably, puts quality and integrity into every batch.

Some herbalists teach - passing on lineage through classes and workshops, writing about plants, developing curricula, mentoring new practitioners. The herbalist-teacher extends their influence through the people they train, creating ripples that spread far beyond what any individual practice could reach.

Some herbalists grow - cultivating medicinal plants, stewarding wild populations, supplying herbs to the community with the care that comes from having tended the plants from seed to harvest. The grower connects people to the earth, to the reality that medicine comes from somewhere, from soil and sun and rain and the patient work of cultivation.

Some herbalists research - studying traditional plant uses, contributing to scientific literature, documenting knowledge that might otherwise be lost, bridging traditional wisdom and modern understanding. The researcher adds to the collective knowledge, asking questions that only careful investigation can answer.

And some herbalists do some blend of these, or something else entirely - integrating plant medicine into another healing modality, focusing on a specific population or condition, developing approaches that don't fit neat categories. Your path need not look like anyone else's. The herbalism the world needs is not uniform but diverse, as diverse as the plants themselves and the people who need their medicine.

What calls you? Not what you think you should do, or what seems practical, or what others are doing -

but what lights up in you when you imagine doing it? Follow that light. It knows something about your path that analysis cannot reveal.

The Gifts You Bring

You do not come to this work empty-handed. You bring everything you are - your life experience, your wounds and your healing from them, your natural gifts, your cultural background, your other skills and trainings, your particular way of seeing the world. All of this shapes the herbalist you become and the contribution you make.

What has your life taught you that informs your herbal practice? Perhaps you've navigated your own health challenges and understand from inside what it is to seek healing. Perhaps you've trained in another field - counseling, bodywork, nutrition, art - that now weaves with your plant knowledge. Perhaps your cultural background connects you to traditional practices that have their own wisdom to offer. Perhaps you have natural gifts of intuition, or analytical thinking, or teaching, or creating beauty, that shape how you work with plants and people.

These gifts are not separate from your herbalism; they are part of it. The herbalist who is also an artist will create medicine and educational materials with aesthetic care that speaks to people differently than plain information would. The herbalist who is also a counselor will hold space for the emotional dimensions of health in ways that others might not. The herbalist who has navigated chronic illness will understand that journey from inside. The herbalist connected to a traditional culture brings that lineage into the present.

Reflect on what you uniquely bring. Not to inflate your ego but to recognize what you have to offer. The world doesn't need another generic herbalist; it needs *you*, with your particular combination of gifts and experiences and perspectives. What only you can offer is what you should most seriously consider offering.

Honoring Lineage

You do not practice in isolation. You stand in lineage - threads of knowledge and relationship extending back through time, connecting you to everyone who has ever worked with these plants and passed on what they learned. The woman who first noticed that chamomile calmed an anxious stomach, the healers who refined understanding through centuries of observation, the teachers who trained your teachers, the authors of books that shaped your learning, the plants themselves who have been teaching humans since humans existed - all of these live in your practice. You are the current expression of a lineage that extends back to the beginning of human relationship with the green world.

Honor this lineage. Acknowledge those who have taught you, directly and through their writings and through the traditions they passed down. Recognize that you know what you know because others took the time to learn it and the care to share it. Feel the weight and the gift of standing in a long line of plant people who have tended this relationship across generations.

Honoring lineage also means passing it forward. What you have received is not yours to hoard but to transmit - through the people you help, the students you teach if you teach, the knowledge you share, the plants you tend and protect. Lineage is a river, not a pond; it flows through you toward those who come after. Your responsibility is to receive it well, add your own experience and understanding, and pass it on with care.

And honoring lineage means practicing with integrity - not claiming what isn't yours, not taking from traditions without respect and permission, not pretending to expertise you haven't earned. Cultural knowledge belongs to the cultures that developed it. Traditional practices deserve acknowledgment of their sources. The humility to give credit, to admit what you don't know, to avoid appropriation - this too is how you honor the lineage you've received.

SACRED RECIPROCITY

From the beginning, we have spoken of reciprocity - the understanding that relationship with plants is not extraction but exchange, not taking but participating in a cycle of giving and receiving. As your practice deepens, reciprocity becomes not just philosophy but lived daily reality.

To the plants, you offer attention and protection. You harvest respectfully, taking only what's needed, never depleting populations. You cultivate medicinal species, expanding their presence rather than diminishing it. You spread seeds. You protect wild places where they grow. You speak for their protection in a world that would pave them over for parking lots. You sit with them in gratitude, acknowledging the gift of their medicine with something more than just taking it.

To the earth that grows them, you offer care. You reduce your consumption. You choose sustainability over convenience. You support conservation. You recognize that every choice you make affects the web of life that includes the plants you love. You vote and advocate and spend your money in ways that protect rather than degrade the living world.

To the human communities you serve, you offer accessibility. You make medicine available to those who need it, not just those who can easily pay. You share knowledge generously. You support those who can't afford conventional healthcare. You respect cultural knowledge and practices. You build community resilience, not just individual health.

To future generations, you offer protection. You safeguard plant populations so they will exist for those not yet born. You pass on knowledge and skills so the lineage continues. You advocate for the future even when the present makes it hard to think beyond immediate needs. You make choices considering not just yourself but those who will inherit what you leave behind.

Reciprocity is not a debt to be paid off but a relationship to be lived. It deepens with practice. Let it become so woven into how you work that you cannot imagine working any other way.

THE HUMILITY OF MASTERY

Here is a paradox: the more you learn, the more you realize how much you don't know. This is not failure; this is wisdom. The beginner often feels confident because they don't know enough to know what they're missing. The master feels humble because they've glimpsed how vast the territory is, how much remains unexplored, how much the plants keep secret even from those who have worked with them for decades.

Practice this humility. Stay in beginner's mind even as your skill grows. Admit when you don't know - to yourself and to those you serve. Refer to practitioners with more experience or different expertise when that serves the person better than your own offering. Learn from everyone: from clients who teach you what your formulas actually do, from plants that reveal new aspects of themselves, from other herbalists who see things you've missed, from research that challenges what you thought you knew.

Be willing to be wrong. Be willing to change your mind when evidence or experience suggests you should. Don't claim expertise you haven't earned or knowledge you don't have. Continue learning always - not as obligation but as joy, the ongoing exploration of a territory that can never be fully mapped.

And respect the mystery. Plants don't give up all their secrets. Bodies heal in ways we don't fully understand. Life itself remains fundamentally mysterious despite all our science. Hold your knowledge loosely, recognizing that it's partial, provisional, always subject to revision by deeper understanding. The best herbalists live in this balance: confident enough in their competence to act, humble enough about their limits to stay curious.

Practical Matters

If you choose to offer herbal services or products beyond your immediate circle, practical matters arise that deserve thoughtful attention. These are not separate from your spiritual and ethical commitments; they are expressions of them.

Know your local laws - what herbalists can legally do in your area, what licensing or registration might be required, what product labeling laws apply, what insurance you might need. These vary significantly by location; learn what applies where you practice. Work within the legal framework while also advocating for changes where the framework unnecessarily limits beneficial practice.

Maintain professional standards - clear scope of practice that you can articulate and honor, informed consent for those you work with, confidentiality about what people share, documentation of your work, continuing education that keeps your knowledge current, professional liability insurance if you're seeing clients.

Consider accessibility. How can you serve those who can't easily pay? Sliding scales, barter arrangements, low-cost community clinics, free educational offerings - these make plant medicine available beyond those with resources. Herbalism has always been medicine of the people; keep it accessible to the people.

Source herbs ethically. Know where your herbs come from. Choose sustainably wildcrafted or organically cultivated herbs. Support suppliers who pay fair prices to growers and harvesters. Avoid herbs that are endangered or threatened unless you can source them from cultivated populations. Your choices as a buyer shape what's available and how it's produced.

Be honest in how you represent what you offer. Don't promise cures. Don't make claims you can't support. Don't pretend to credentials you don't have. Let your integrity be so evident that those who work with you trust you completely - because you've earned that trust by being trustworthy.

The Work Continues

This book is foundation, not completion. The path of the herbalist continues as long as you continue walking it.

Continue your education. Study with master herbalists who can take you deeper than books alone. Pursue advanced training in areas that call you - clinical practice, formulation, specific body systems, traditional systems like Chinese medicine or Ayurveda. Learn related fields that complement your herbal knowledge: nutrition, anatomy and physiology, counseling skills, botany and plant identification, cultivation and wildcrafting.

Continue your direct plant study. Spend time with plants in their habitats. Grow medicinal herbs if you can - nothing teaches you a plant like tending it from seed to harvest. Wildcraft responsibly, deepening your identification skills and your understanding of plant communities. Learn from Indigenous and traditional practitioners where such learning is offered respectfully and with permission.

Continue building community. Join professional organizations. Attend conferences and gatherings. Participate in plant walks and workshops. Build relationships with other herbalists. Find or create study groups. The path is less lonely when walked with others, and the field benefits from practitioners who support each other.

And practice. See people - starting with friends and family, expanding as your skill grows. Document your work and learn from each case. Volunteer at herbal clinics if they exist in your area. Work alongside more experienced practitioners when possible. There is no substitute for practice; it's where everything you've learned meets reality and transforms into lived skill.

Embodied Practice: The Alchemist's Dedication

This final practice is not a technique to learn but a ceremony to enact - a formal marking of the threshold you have crossed and the commitment you carry forward. It is both completion of what you have done and consecration of what you will do. Create it with the care it deserves.

You'll need time and space where you won't be interrupted. Representatives of your practice - perhaps a few key herbs from your materia medica, your journal, medicines you have made. A candle or other flame. Something to write with and something to write on that you can keep. And your full presence, your willingness to mark this moment as the threshold it is.

Prepare the Space

Create a space that feels sacred to you - whatever that means in your tradition and understanding. Perhaps you cleanse the space with smoke or sound or simply with intention. Perhaps you call in directions or guides or simply quiet yourself. Arrange your materials: the herbs, the journal, the medicines, the candle unlit, the writing materials. Let the arrangement itself be intentional, creating a form that holds the ceremony.

When the space is ready, sit quietly and let yourself arrive. Breathe. Feel your body, the floor beneath you, the air around you. Let the busy mind settle. You are about to mark something significant; let yourself be fully present for it.

ACKNOWLEDGE WHAT HAS BEEN

Light the candle. As you do, acknowledge the journey you have made. Not in detail but in essence: you came seeking, you studied, you practiced, you were changed. Speak aloud if that feels right - acknowledging the teachers who have guided you (present and past, human and plant), the challenges you faced and moved through, the transformation that has occurred in you.

Pick up each of the herbs you've gathered, one at a time. For each, acknowledge your relationship - how you met this plant, what it has taught you, what you appreciate about it. Let yourself feel gratitude for these plant allies who have become part of your life and practice. Don't rush; let each acknowledgment be real.

If you've brought medicines you made, hold them. Acknowledge what went into their creation - the plants, your skill, the intention, the alchemical transformation from raw material to refined medicine. Let yourself feel the accomplishment of what you've learned to create.

DECLARE WHO YOU HAVE BECOME

Now, write your declaration - a statement of who you are as an herbalist and how you will practice. This is not a business plan or a resume; it's a statement of identity and commitment. Write from your heart, not your strategic mind. You might include: what you understand your work to be, what values guide your practice, what gifts you bring, what populations or issues call you, what you commit to in terms of ethics and reciprocity and continued growth.

Write until you feel complete. Then read what you've written aloud - to yourself, to the plants gathered with you, to whatever forces or guides you recognize. Let the words be spoken into the world. This is your declaration of identity, your statement of becoming. *I am an herbalist, and this is how I will practice.*

RECEIVE THE COMMITMENT

Sit in silence after reading your declaration. Let it settle. Feel what it feels like to have spoken these words, to have named who you are and how you will practice. Notice what arises - perhaps pride, perhaps humility, perhaps excitement or fear or both. Let whatever arises be present without needing to change it.

Imagine the lineage you stand in - the long line of plant people extending back through time. Imagine them hearing your declaration, welcoming you into their company, acknowledging that you have done the work and are ready to carry it forward. You are not alone in this work; you join a vast community of those who have tended the relationship between humans and healing plants.

Close the Ceremony

When you feel ready, close the ceremony in whatever way is right for you. Perhaps thanks to the guides or directions you called in. Perhaps simply a breath and a bow. Extinguish the candle with intention, acknowledging that the ceremony is complete but the work continues.

Keep your written declaration somewhere you can return to it - in your journal, on your altar, in a special place. Let it remind you of who you are and what you've committed to. Return to it when you need grounding, when you've lost your way, when you need to remember why you do this work.

You have marked the threshold. You have named yourself. Now: go forth and practice.

Reflection Questions

1. Looking back at who you were when you began this journey, what has changed? What transformation do you recognize in yourself?

2. What kind of herbalist are you becoming? What path calls to you most clearly?

3. What unique gifts do you bring to this work? What can you offer that only you can offer?

4. What lineage do you honor? What traditions have shaped you, and how will you honor and transmit what you've received?

5. How will you practice reciprocity in concrete ways? What will you give back to plants, to earth, to community, to future generations?

6. What is your growing edge - the place where you're still developing, still learning, still uncertain? How will you tend that edge with both confidence and humility?

Closing Words

You crossed the threshold as seeker. You learned to listen to plants, to taste their wisdom on your tongue, to recognize their signatures and actions and affinities. You mastered the alchemical languages of preparation - transforming crude plant matter into refined medicine through water and alcohol and honey and heat and time. You learned to read bodies, to recognize the patterns written in tissue and constitution, to match plant to person with growing skill. You followed the seasons and absorbed their wisdom. You walked with the moon. You created formulas from relationship.

Now you stand here: transformed.

You are not just someone who knows about herbs. You are not just someone who can make medicine or offer recommendations. You are an herbalist - a person who has entered the ancient compact between humans and healing plants, who has received the lineage and carries it forward, who has been changed by the plants and continues to be changed, who offers themselves as vessel through which healing can occur.

The plants have been waiting for you to remember this truth: you are not separate from them. You are not their master, their owner, their exploiter. You are not even, truly, their student - or rather, you are student and they are student too, both of you learning each other, both of you changed by the relationship. You are family. You belong to each other.

Go forth with competence born of rigorous study and practice. Go forth with humility born of knowing how much you don't know and how vast the territory remains. Go forth with joy - because this work is joyful, because relationship with plants is joyful, because helping people find their way toward balance is joyful. Go forth with commitment to reciprocity and ethics, to honoring lineage, to protecting the plants and the earth that grows them. Go forth with wonder at the mystery that remains, the secrets the plants still keep, the depths you have not yet plumbed.

The world needs your medicine. Not because you are special - though you are - but because the world needs medicine and you have learned to make it. People are suffering. Bodies are out of balance.

The medical system fails to serve many. The plants are waiting to help, and they need human allies to make their medicine available. You have made yourself such an ally.

Go forth as yourself, fully. Practice with integrity. Stay humble. Keep learning. Remember reciprocity always. Honor lineage. Be the alchemist, craft the medicine.

Welcome to the path. The journey continues forever.

The plants are waiting.
The world needs your medicine.

Glossary of Herbs

This glossary offers a quick reference to the herbs discussed throughout this book. Each entry includes the common name, Latin binomial, primary actions, and the chapter(s) where the herb is explored in depth. This is intended as a navigational aid, not a substitute for the fuller discussions in each chapter or for your own developing materia medica.

A

Artichoke *(Cynara scolymus)* — Bitter, cholagogue, hepatoprotective. Stimulates bile flow and supports liver function. Chapter 5

Ashwagandha *(Withania somnifera)* — Adaptogen, nervine tonic, anti-inflammatory. Calms while building energy; specific for 'wired but tired' patterns. Warm, grounding. Chapters 7, 8, 10

Astragalus *(Astragalus membranaceus)* — Immune modulator, adaptogen, tonic. Builds deep immune resilience over time; safe for long-term use. Warm, sweet. Chapter 6

B

Black Cohosh *(Actaea racemosa)* — Hormone modulator, anti-inflammatory, antispasmodic. Specific for menopausal symptoms, especially hot flashes. Cooling. Chapters 8, 10

Burdock *(Arctium lappa)* — Alterative, nutritive, lymphatic. Gentle blood cleanser supporting liver and skin; root is mildly sweet and grounding. Chapter 5

C

Calendula *(Calendula officinalis)* — Lymphatic, vulnerary, anti-inflammatory, antimicrobial. Heals tissue inside and out; moves lymph gently. Cooling. Chapters 5, 9

Chamomile *(Matricaria chamomilla)* — Nervine relaxant, carminative, anti-inflammatory, bitter. Gentle enough for children and elders; calms digestion and nerves simultaneously. Cooling. Chapters 5, 7, 9, 10

Cleavers *(Galium aparine)* — Lymphatic, diuretic, alterative. Premier lymph mover; cooling and cleansing. Best used fresh or as fresh plant tincture. Chapter 5

Cramp Bark *(Viburnum opulus)* — Antispasmodic, nervine. Relaxes smooth and skeletal muscle; specific for menstrual cramps. Chapter 8

D

Dandelion *(Taraxacum officinale)* — Bitter, cholagogue, diuretic, nutritive. Root supports liver; leaf is potassium-sparing diuretic. Cooling. Chapters 5, 10

Dong Quai *(Angelica sinensis)* — Blood tonic, uterine tonic, circulatory. Nourishes and builds blood; traditionally used in formulas rather than alone. Warm, moistening. Chapter 8

E

Echinacea *(Echinacea purpurea, E. angustifolia)* — Immune stimulant, antimicrobial, lymphatic. For acute infection; use intensively and short-term. Quality crucial—should tingle on tongue. Chapter 6

Elderberry *(Sambucus nigra)* — Immune stimulant, antiviral, diaphoretic. Specific for flu; must be cooked (raw berries toxic). Cooling. Chapter 6

Elderflower *(Sambucus nigra)* — Diaphoretic, anticatarrhal, relaxant. Opens pores to release fever; dries excess mucus. Cooling. Chapter 6

Elecampane *(Inula helenium)* — Expectorant, antimicrobial, bitter. For deep, stuck lung congestion; warming and moving. Chapter 6

Eucalyptus *(Eucalyptus globulus)* — Antimicrobial, expectorant, decongestant. Opens airways; best used as steam inhalation or chest rub. Cooling, strongly aromatic. Chapter 6

Eyebright *(Euphrasia officinalis)* — Anticatarrhal, anti-inflammatory, astringent. Specific for eyes and upper respiratory; drying. Chapter 6

F

Fennel *(Foeniculum vulgare)* — Carminative, antispasmodic, galactagogue. Releases trapped gas; eases digestive cramping. Warm, sweet. Chapters 5, 10

G

Garlic *(Allium sativum)* — Antimicrobial, hypotensive, antiplatelet, immune stimulant. Cardiovascular support; potent when raw. Hot, pungent. Chapter 6

Gentian *(Gentiana lutea)* — Bitter, digestive stimulant. One of the most bitter herbs; small amounts stimulate entire digestive cascade. Very cooling. Chapter 5

Ginger *(Zingiber officinale)* — Carminative, circulatory stimulant, antiemetic, anti-inflammatory. Warms digestion, activates formulas, eases nausea. Hot, pungent. Chapters 5, 6, 7, 8, 10

Goldenrod *(Solidago spp.)* — Anticatarrhal, anti-inflammatory, astringent, diuretic. Upper respiratory and urinary support; drying. Chapter 6

Gotu Kola *(Centella asiatica)* — Nervine tonic, cognitive support, vulnerary. Supports nerve regeneration and mental clarity. Cooling. Chapter 7

H

Hawthorn *(Crataegus spp.)* — Cardiotonic, hypotensive, antioxidant. Strengthens heart over time; also for emotional heart. Effects gradual—use for months. Chapter 6

Holy Basil / Tulsi *(Ocimum sanctum)* — Adaptogen, nervine, immunomodulator. Uplifting while building reserves; balances blood sugar. Warm, aromatic. Chapter 8

Horehound *(Marrubium vulgare)* — Expectorant, bitter, antispasmodic. For productive coughs; very bitter. Chapter 6

Horsetail *(Equisetum arvense)* — Astringent, diuretic, connective tissue support. Highest plant source of silica; use in cycles (6 weeks on, 2 off). Chapter 7

L

Lavender *(Lavandula angustifolia)* — Nervine relaxant, carminative, antimicrobial. Calming; specific for tension headaches. Cooling, aromatic. Chapters 7, 10

Lemon Balm *(Melissa officinalis)* — Nervine relaxant, carminative, antiviral. Uplifting and calming simultaneously; supports digestion. Cooling. Chapters 7, 9, 10

Licorice *(Glycyrrhiza glabra)* — Demulcent, adaptogen, harmonizer, adrenal support. Unifies formulas; soothes mucous membranes. Use caution with hypertension. Chapters 6, 8, 10

M

Marshmallow *(Althaea officinalis)* — Demulcent, vulnerary, emollient. Soothes and protects irritated tissue; root for digestion, leaf for urinary/respiratory. Cool, moist. Chapters 6, 10

Milk Thistle *(Silybum marianum)* — Hepatoprotective, antioxidant, cholagogue. Protects and regenerates liver cells; seeds most potent. Chapter 5

Milky Oat Tops *(Avena sativa)* — Nervine tonic, nutritive, restorative. Supreme nervous system rebuilder; must be harvested in 'milky' stage for full potency. Chapters 7, 8, 10

Motherwort *(Leonurus cardiaca)* — Nervine, cardiac tonic, emmenagogue. Calms anxiety with heart palpitations; specific for menopausal transition. Cooling, bitter. Chapters 8, 10

Mullein *(Verbascum thapsus)* — Demulcent, expectorant, anti-inflammatory. Soothes dry, irritated respiratory tissue. Must strain well (tiny hairs). Cool, moist. Chapter 6

N

Nettles *(Urtica dioica)* — Nutritive, alterative, anti-inflammatory, diuretic. Mineral-rich; supports bones, blood, allergies. Long-steep infusions extract minerals. Chapters 5, 7, 8, 10

O

Oatstraw *(Avena sativa)* — Nutritive, nervine (mild), demulcent. Dried stalks and leaves; mineral-rich, gentle nervous system support. Distinct from milky oat tops. Chapters 7, 8

Oregano *(Origanum vulgare)* — Antimicrobial, expectorant, carminative. Strong respiratory antimicrobial; warming and drying. Chapter 6

P

Passionflower *(Passiflora incarnata)* — Nervine relaxant, sedative, anxiolytic, antispasmodic. For circular/obsessive thoughts preventing sleep; works on GABA pathways. Cooling. Chapters 7, 10

Peppermint *(Mentha × piperita)* — Carminative, antispasmodic, mild stimulant, antimicrobial. Alerting and cooling; eases digestive cramping. Chapter 7

R

Raspberry Leaf *(Rubus idaeus)* — Uterine tonic, astringent, nutritive. Tones uterine muscle; traditional for pregnancy and menstrual support. Mineral-rich. Chapter 8

Red Clover *(Trifolium pratense)* — Alterative, lymphatic, nutritive, phytoestrogenic. Gentle clearing; bone and menopausal support. Caution with hormone-sensitive conditions. Chapters 5, 7, 8

Reishi *(Ganoderma lucidum)* — Immunomodulator, adaptogen, nervine, hepatoprotective. 'Mushroom of immortality'; nourishes spirit, supports sleep. Bitter. Chapter 8

Rosemary *(Salvia rosmarinus)* — Circulatory stimulant, nervine stimulant, antioxidant. Mental clarity and memory; warming and aromatic. Chapter 7

S

Sage *(Salvia officinalis)* — Astringent, antimicrobial, carminative, reduces sweating. Specific for night sweats and hot flashes. Drying. Chapters 6, 8, 10

Shatavari *(Asparagus racemosus)* — Adaptogen, reproductive tonic, demulcent. Nourishing for female reproductive system; cooling, moistening counterpart to ashwagandha. Chapter 8

Shepherd's Purse *(Capsella bursa-pastoris)* — Astringent, hemostatic. Strong astringent for acute heavy bleeding. Chapter 8

Skullcap *(Scutellaria lateriflora)* — Nervine relaxant and tonic, antispasmodic. Calms racing thoughts; both acute relief and long-term support. Cool, bitter. Quality crucial. Chapters 7, 8, 10

Slippery Elm *(Ulmus rubra)* — Demulcent, nutritive, vulnerary. Soothes entire digestive tract; sustainably sourced inner bark only. Cool, moist. Chapter 6

St. John's Wort *(Hypericum perforatum)* — Nervine tonic, antidepressant, vulnerary, antiviral. Mood support; topically for nerve pain. Many drug interactions—check carefully. Chapter 7

T

Thyme *(Thymus vulgaris)* — Antimicrobial, expectorant, antispasmodic, carminative. Broad-spectrum respiratory antimicrobial. Warm, aromatic. Cover while steeping. Chapter 6

V

Valerian *(Valeriana officinalis)* — Nervine relaxant, sedative, antispasmodic. Powerful sedation for sleep; not subtle. Warm. Some find it stimulating—individual variation. Chapters 7, 10

Vitex / Chaste Tree Berry *(Vitex agnus-castus)* — Hormone modulator. Acts on pituitary to support progesterone; for PMS, irregular cycles, fertility. Takes 3-6 months; not during pregnancy. Chapter 8

W

Wild Cherry Bark *(Prunus serotina)* — Antitussive, astringent, sedative. Calms dry, irritating coughs. Use in moderation; contains compounds that break down to cyanide in large amounts. Chapter 6

Wood Betony *(Stachys officinalis)* — Nervine, bitter, circulatory. Grounding; clears mental fog, tension headaches. Chapter 7

Y

Yarrow *(Achillea millefolium)* — Diaphoretic, astringent, bitter, styptic, anti-inflammatory. Versatile; moves blood, stops bleeding, opens pores for fever. Cooling, drying. Chapters 5, 8

Yellow Dock *(Rumex crispus)* — Alterative, bitter, mild laxative, iron-enhancing. Supports liver and gentle elimination; helps iron absorption. Chapter 5

A Note on This Glossary

This glossary represents a beginning, not a completion. The herbs listed here are those explored within this book, but the plant kingdom offers thousands more allies awaiting relationship. As your practice deepens, you will meet new plants and add them to your personal materia medica.

Remember that brief descriptions cannot capture the fullness of any plant's medicine. Each herb listed here is a living being with its own intelligence, its own complexity, its own gifts that reveal themselves only through direct relationship over time. Use this glossary as a quick reference, but let your real knowledge come from the plants themselves—from growing them, harvesting them, preparing them, tasting them, working with them, and learning from the results.

The best materia medica is the one you build yourself, from your own experience, in your own hand.

About the Author

Dr. Stephanie Shelburne is a visionary thought-leader for individual and global coherence, and a practitioner of Mind-Body Medicine, Holistic Nutrition, and Somatic Psychology. Her work bridges the mythic and the Monday morning - weaving scientific rigor with embodied wisdom to help people access the intelligence that lives in their bones. Through her Sacred Metabolism framework, she guides women beyond the "fix-it" paradigm into a deeper honoring of the body's sophisticated wisdom. She lives on a farm in Vermont, surrounded by the animals and plants who continue to be her greatest teachers.

www.drstephanieshelburne.com

The New England School of Bioenergetic Medicine

NESBEM is an educational institution dedicated to creating a coherence movement for humans, non-humans, and the planet. We offer transformative programs that bridge Western biomedical science with traditional healing wisdom, cultivating practitioners who are as grounded in research as they are in relationship with the living world. Our approach honors the body's innate intelligence, the sovereignty of plants, and the interconnected web of life that makes healing possible.

www.newenglandschoolbem.org

Continue the Journey

This book is a threshold. If you are ready to walk through it with guidance, community, and deep practice, we invite you to join our **Integrative Herbal Medicine Program** - a ten-module journey based on the teachings in these pages. Over the course of the program, you will build your own materia medica through direct relationship with plants, develop clinical thinking and formulation skills, and undergo the alchemical transformation from seeker to practitioner.

This is not passive learning. It is an apprenticeship - elemental, primal, and guided every step of the way. You will taste, prepare, observe, create, and be changed. By the program's end, you will not only know the plants; you will have become an herbalist.

The plants are waiting. The community is gathering.

Will you join us?

www.newenglandschoolbem.org/integrative-herbal-medicine